Advances in Atrial Fibrillation Ablation

Editors

LUIGI DI BIASE
FRANCIS MARCHLINSKI
ANDREA NATALE

CARDIAC ELECTROPHYSIOLOGY CLINICS

www.cardiacEP.theclinics.com

Consulting Editors
RANJAN K. THAKUR
ANDREA NATALE

June 2020 • Volume 12 • Number 2

ELSEVIER

1600 John F. Kennedy Boulevard • Suite 1800 • Philadelphia, Pennsylvania, 19103-2899

http://www.theclinics.com

CARDIAC ELECTROPHYSIOLOGY CLINICS Volume 12, Number 2
June 2020 ISSN 1877-9182, ISBN-13: 978-0-323-76199-4

Editor: Stacy Eastman
Developmental Editor: Donald Mumford

Cardiac Electrophysiology Clinics (ISSN 1877-9182) is published quarterly by Elsevier Inc., 360 Park Avenue South, New York, NY 10010-1710. Months of issue are March, June, September, and December. Subscription prices are $231.00 per year for US individuals, $388.00 per year for US institutions, $249.00 per year for Canadian individuals, $438.00 per year for Canadian institutions, $303.00 per year for international individuals, $469.00 per year for international institutions and $100.00 per year for US, Canadian and international students/residents. To receive student/resident rate, orders must be accompanied by name of affiliated institution, date of term, and the signature of program/residency coordinator on institution letterhead. Orders will be billed at individual rate until proof of status is received. Foreign air speed delivery is included in all Clinics subscription prices. All prices are subject to change without notice. **POSTMASTER:** Send address changes to Cardiac Electrophysiology Clinics, Elsevier Health Sciences Division, Subscription Customer Service, 3251 Riverport Lane, Maryland Heights, MO 63043. **Customer Service: 1-800-654-2452 (US and Canada). From outside of the US and Canada, call 314-477-8871. Fax: 314-447-8029. E-mail: JournalsCustomerService-usa@elsevier.com (for print support); JournalsOnlineSupport-usa@elsevier.com (for online support).**

Reprints. For copies of 100 or more of articles in this publication, please contact the Commercial Reprints Department, Elsevier Inc., 360 Park Avenue South, New York, NY 10010-1710. Tel.: 212-633-3874; Fax: 212-633-3820; E-mail: reprints@elsevier.com.

Cardiac Electrophysiology Clinics is covered in MEDLINE/PubMed (Index Medicus).

Contributors

CONSULTING EDITORS

RANJAN K. THAKUR, MD, MPH, MBA, FHRS
Professor of Medicine and Director, Arrhythmia
Service, Thoracic and Cardiovascular Institute,
Sparrow Health System, Michigan State
University, Lansing, Michigan, USA

ANDREA NATALE, MD, FACC, FHRS
Executive Medical Director of the Texas
Cardiac Arrhythmia Institute, St. David's
Medical Center, Austin, Texas, Professor, Dell

Medical School, University of Texas at Austin,
Austin, Texas, USA; National Medical Director,
Cardiac Electrophysiology, California,
Consulting Professor, Division of Cardiology,
Stanford University, California, USA; Clinical
Professor of Medicine, Case Western Reserve
University, Cleveland, Ohio, USA; Director,
Interventional Electrophysiology, Scripps
Clinic, San Diego, California, USA

EDITORS

LUIGI DI BIASE, MD, PhD, FACC, FHRS
Professor of Medicine, Department of
Medicine (Cardiology), Section Head
Electrophysiology, Director of Arrhythmia
Services, Albert Einstein College of Medicine,
Montefiore Hospital, Montefiore-Einstein
Center for Heart and Vascular Care, New York,
New York, USA

FRANCIS MARCHLINSKI, MD, FACC, FHRS
Richard T and Angela Clark President's
Distinguished Professor of Medicine, Director
of Electrophysiology, University of
Pennsylvania Health System, Director of
Electrophysiology Laboratory, Hospital of the
University of Pennsylvania, Perelman School of

Medicine, University of Pennsylvania,
Philadelphia, Pennsylvania, USA

ANDREA NATALE, MD, FACC, FHRS
Executive Medical Director of the Texas
Cardiac Arrhythmia Institute, St. David's
Medical Center, Austin, Texas, Professor, Dell
Medical School, University of Texas at Austin,
Austin, Texas, USA; National Medical Director,
Cardiac Electrophysiology, California,
Consulting Professor, Division of Cardiology,
Stanford University, California, USA; Clinical
Professor of Medicine, Case Western
Reserve University, Cleveland, Ohio, USA;
Director, Interventional Electrophysiology,
Scripps Clinic, San Diego, California, USA

AUTHORS

BRYAN MAC DONALD, MD
Texas Cardiac Arrhythmia Institute, St. David's
Medical Center, Austin, Texas, USA

ISABELLA ALVIZ, MD
Montefiore-Einstein Center for Heart and
Vascular Care, Montefiore Medical Center,

Albert Einstein College of Medicine, New York,
New York, USA

ALISARA ANANNAB, MD
Texas Cardiac Arrhythmia Institute, St. David's
Medical Center, Austin, Texas, USA;
Electrophysiology Unit, Department of

Cardiovascular Interventions, Central Chest Institute of Thailand, Nonthaburi, Thailand

JONATHAN P. ARIYARATNAM, MB BChir
Centre for Heart Rhythm Disorders, University of Adelaide, Royal Adelaide Hospital, Adelaide, South Australia, Australia

ARASH ARYANA, MD, PhD, FACC, FHRS
Medical Director, Cardiovascular Services Mercy General Hospital, Dignity Health Heart and Vascular Institute, Sacramento, California, USA

RAHUL BHARDWAJ, MD
Assistant Professor, Loma Linda University, Loma Linda, California, USA

DAVID F. BRICEÑO, MD
Montefiore-Einstein Center for Heart and Vascular Care, Montefiore Medical Center, Albert Einstein College of Medicine, New York, New York, USA

HUGH CALKINS, MD
Professor of Medicine, Division of Cardiology, Section for Cardiac Electrophysiology, Johns Hopkins University, Baltimore, Maryland, USA

DAVID J. CALLANS, MD
Professor of Medicine, Cardiovascular Division, Electrophysiology Section, Hospital of the University of Pennsylvania, Philadelphia, Pennsylvania, USA

THARIAN S. CHERIAN, MD
Electrophysiology Fellow, Cardiovascular Division, Electrophysiology Section, Hospital of the University of Pennsylvania, Philadelphia, Pennsylvania, USA

GIAN-BATTISTA CHIERCHIA, MD, PhD
Heart Rhythm Management Center, UZ Brussel–VUB, Brussels, Belgium

JONATHAN CHRISPIN, MD
Assistant Professor of Medicine, Division of Cardiology, Section for Cardiac Electrophysiology, Johns Hopkins University, Baltimore, Maryland, USA

CARLO DE ASMUNDIS, MD, PhD
Heart Rhythm Management Center, UZ Brussel–VUB, Brussels, Belgium

DOMENICO G. DELLA ROCCA, MD
Texas Cardiac Arrhythmia Institute, St. David's Medical Center, Austin, Texas, USA

LUIGI DI BIASE, MD, PhD, FACC, FHRS
Professor of Medicine, Department of Medicine (Cardiology), Section Head Electrophysiology, Director of Arrhythmia Services, Albert Einstein College of Medicine, Montefiore Hospital, Montefiore-Einstein Center for Heart and Vascular Care, New York, New York, USA

SRINIVAS R. DUKKIPATI, MD
Associate Professor, Mount Sinai School of Medicine, New York, New York, USA

DAVID S. FRANKEL, MD
Associate Professor of Medicine, Fellowship Director, Section of Cardiac Electrophysiology, Division of Cardiovascular Medicine, Perelman School of Medicine at the University of Pennsylvania, Philadelphia, Pennsylvania, USA

CAROLA GIANNI, MD
Texas Cardiac Arrhythmia Institute, St. David's Medical Center, Austin, Texas, USA

MOHAMMADALI HABIBI, MD
Cardiac Electrophysiology Fellow, Division of Cardiology, Section for Cardiac Electrophysiology, Johns Hopkins University, Baltimore, Maryland, USA

HENRY HALPERIN, MD, PhD
Professor of Medicine, Division of Cardiology, Section for Cardiac Electrophysiology, Department of Biomedical Engineering, Johns Hopkins University, Baltimore, Maryland, USA

SURAJ KAPA, MD, FHRS
Associate Professor of Medicine, Department of Cardiovascular Medicine, Mayo Clinic, Rochester, Minnesota, USA

SANTHISRI KODALI, MD
Assistant Professor of Medicine, Cardiac Electrophysiology, The University of Texas Medical Branch, Galveston, Texas, USA

JACOB S. KORUTH, MD
Assistant Professor, Mount Sinai School of Medicine, New York, New York, USA

GURUKRIPA N. KOWLGI, MBBS, MD
Department of Cardiovascular Medicine, Mayo
Clinic, Rochester, Minnesota, USA

DENNIS LAU, MBBS, PhD
Associate Professor, Centre for Heart Rhythm
Disorders, University of Adelaide, Royal
Adelaide Hospital, Adelaide, South Australia,
Australia

ANGEL QUINTERO MAYEDO, MD
Texas Cardiac Arrhythmia Institute, St. David's
Medical Center, Austin, Texas, USA

MELISSA MIDDELDORP, PhD
Centre for Heart Rhythm Disorders, University
of Adelaide, Royal Adelaide Hospital, Adelaide,
South Australia, Australia

SANGHAMITRA MOHANTY, MD
Texas Cardiac Arrhythmia Institute, St. David's
Medical Center, Dell Medical School,
University of Texas, Austin, Texas, USA

ANDREA NATALE, MD, FACC, FHRS
Executive Medical Director of the Texas
Cardiac Arrhythmia Institute, St. David's
Medical Center, Austin, Texas, Professor,
Dell Medical School, University of Texas at
Austin, Austin, Texas, USA; National Medical
Director, Cardiac Electrophysiology,
California, Consulting Professor, Division of
Cardiology, Stanford University, California,
USA; Clinical Professor of Medicine, Case
Western Reserve University, Cleveland, Ohio,
USA; Director, Interventional
Electrophysiology, Scripps Clinic, San Diego,
California, USA

VERONICA NATALE
Texas Cardiac Arrhythmia Institute, St. David's
Medical Center, Austin, Texas, USA

SAMAN NAZARIAN, MD, PhD
Associate Professor of Medicine, Division of
Cardiology, Section for Cardiac
Electrophysiology, Perelman School of
Medicine, University of Pennsylvania,
Philadelphia, Pennsylvania, USA

PETR NEUZIL, MD, PhD
Homolka Hospital, Prague, Czech Republic

JEAN JACQUES NOUBIAP, MD
Centre for Heart Rhythm Disorders, University
of Adelaide, Royal Adelaide Hospital, Adelaide,
South Australia, Australia

KAVISHA PATEL, MD
Montefiore-Einstein Center for Heart and
Vascular Care, Montefiore Medical Center,
Albert Einstein College of Medicine, New York,
New York, USA

NAGA VENKATA K. POTHINENI, MD
Fellow, Section of Cardiac Electrophysiology,
Division of Cardiovascular Medicine, Perelman
School of Medicine University of Pennsylvania,
Philadelphia, Pennsylvania, USA

VIVEK Y. REDDY, MD
Professor of Medicine, Icahn School of
Medicine at Mount Sinai, New York, New York,
USA

JORGE ROMERO, MD
Montefiore-Einstein Center for Heart and
Vascular Care, Montefiore Medical Center,
Albert Einstein College of Medicine, New York,
New York, USA

ANU SALWAN, MD
Texas Cardiac Arrhythmia Institute, St. David's
Medical Center, Austin, Texas, USA

PRASHANTHAN SANDERS, MBBS, PhD
Professor, Director, Centre for Heart Rhythm
Disorders, University of Adelaide and Royal
Adelaide Hospital, Adelaide, South Australia,
Australia

PASQUALE SANTANGELI, MD, PhD
Associate Professor of Medicine, Cardiac
Electrophysiology, Hospital of the University of
Pennsylvania, Philadelphia, Pennsylvania, USA

DAVID D. SPRAGG, MD
Associate Professor of Medicine, Division of
Cardiology, Section for Cardiac
Electrophysiology, Johns Hopkins University,
Baltimore, Maryland, USA

HARIKRISHNA TANDRI, MD
Associate Professor of Medicine, Division of
Cardiology, Section for Cardiac
Electrophysiology, Johns Hopkins University,
Baltimore, Maryland, USA

NICOLA TARANTINO, MD
Montefiore-Einstein Center for Heart and
Vascular Care, Montefiore Medical Center,
Albert Einstein College of Medicine, New York,
New York, USA

GIJO THOMAS, PhD
Centre for Heart Rhythm Disorders,
University of Adelaide, South Australian
Health and Medical Research Institute
(SAHMRI) Adelaide, South Australia,
Australia

NATALIA TRAYANOVA, PhD
Professor, Department of Biomedical
Engineering, Johns Hopkins University,
Baltimore, Maryland, USA

CHINTAN TRIVEDI, MD
Texas Cardiac Arrhythmia Institute,
St. David's Medical Center, Austin,
Texas, USA

XIAO-DONG ZHANG, MD
Montefiore-Einstein Center for Heart and
Vascular Care, Montefiore Medical Center,
Albert Einstein College of Medicine,
New York, New York, USA

STEFAN L. ZIMMERMAN, MD
Associate Professor, Department of Radiology,
Johns Hopkins University, Baltimore,
Maryland, USA

Contents

Advances in cardiac magnetic resonance (CMR) techniques and image acquisition have made it an excellent tool in the assessment of atrial myopathy. Remolding of the left atrium is the mainstay of atrial fibrillation (AF) development and its progression. CMR can detect phasic atrial volumes, atrial function, and atrial fibrosis using cine, and contrast-enhanced or non–contrast-enhanced images. These abilities make CMR a versatile and extraordinary tool in management of patients with AF including for risk stratification, ablation prognostication and planning, and assessment of stroke risk. We review the latest advancements in utility of CMR in management of patients with AF.

Atrial fibrillation (AF) is increasingly recognized as the cardiac electrophysiologic manifestation of a multifactorial systemic disease. Several risk factors for development of AF have been identified; many are modifiable. There is evidence to suggest that aggressive management of modifiable risk factors has potential to significantly reduce the burden of AF, before and after AF ablation. Specific risk factor management (RFM) clinics have been shown effective in conferring these benefits into tangible improvements in large cohorts of patients. This review discusses the evidence behind RFM as a key adjunctive management strategy alongside AF ablation and suggests a model for RFM in clinics.

High-density (HD) mapping presents opportunities to enhance delineation of atrial fibrillation (AF) substrate, improve efficiency of the mapping procedure without sacrificing safety, and afford new mechanistic insights regarding AF. Innovations in hardware, software algorithms, and development of novel multielectrode catheters have allowed HD mapping to be feasible and reliable. Patients to particularly benefit from this technology are those with paroxysmal AF in setting of preexisting atrial scar, persistent AF, and AF in the setting of complex congenital heart disease. The future will bring refinements in automated HD mapping including evolution of noncontact methodologies and artificial intelligence to supplant current techniques.

mixed. Avoiding ablation on the esophagus with esophageal deviation and modifying ablation approaches may decrease the risk of injury.

Discontinuing Anticoagulation After Catheter Ablation of Atrial Fibrillation

Naga Venkata K. Pothineni and David S. Frankel

Atrial fibrillation is a leading cause of ischemic stroke. Stroke risk can be reduced with oral anticoagulation. Current guidelines recommend that decisions regarding anticoagulation after catheter ablation be based solely on preprocedural risk, as defined by established risk scores. Whether the absolute risk of stroke is sufficiently reduced by successful catheter ablation such that the benefit in terms of further reduction in strokes with continued anticoagulation is outweighed by increased bleeds, remains to be determined. Here, we review the observational data pertaining to anticoagulation discontinuation after atrial fibrillation ablation and describe the authors' practice in this regard.

CARDIAC ELECTROPHYSIOLOGY CLINICS

THE CLINICS ARE AVAILABLE ONLINE!
Access your subscription at:
www.theclinics.com

Foreword
Advances in Atrial Fibrillation Ablation

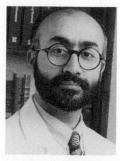

Ranjan K. Thakur, MD, MPH, MBA, FHRS
Consulting Editor

I am pleased to introduce this issue of *Cardiac Electrophysiology Clinics* focused on advances in atrial fibrillation (AF) ablation.

Pulmonary vein–triggered AF was discovered serendipitously by Haissaguerre over 20 years ago. Ablation of these foci became an obvious target, and this has been the focus of clinical and scientific research in cardiac electrophysiology for the last two decades.

We have been successful to a large extent after trying many approaches, but we have not been able to eliminate this problem. We have made many advances. Technological breakthroughs have come and gone, and new ones are still emerging. Many limitations have become apparent, and it has dawned on us that AF is not "curable" in most patients, but it can be palliated to a significant extent. Despite the intense focus on this problem, much remains to be learned.

It is appropriate to take stock at this juncture. We will not be able to summarize the entire field and therefore focus our discussion on promising ideas that are at the forefront at this time. I congratulate Drs Di Biase, Marchlinski, and Natale, the editors of this issue, for selecting topics that are of interest to the readership and getting thought-leaders to concisely pen contemporary thinking.

I hope the readership will enjoy reading these timely reviews.

Ranjan K. Thakur, MD, MPH, MBA, FHRS
Sparrow Thoracic and Cardiovascular Institute
Michigan State University
1440 East Michigan Avenue; Suite 400
Lansing, MI 48912, USA

E-mail address:
thakur@msu.edu

Card Electrophysiol Clin 12 (2020) xiii
https://doi.org/10.1016/j.ccep.2020.04.001
1877-9182/20/© 2020 Published by Elsevier Inc.

Preface

Advances in Atrial Fibrillation Ablation

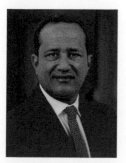

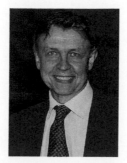

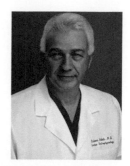

Luigi Di Biase, MD, PhD, FACC, FHRS   Francis Marchlinski, MD, FACC, FHRS   Andrea Natale, MD, FACC, FHRS

Editors

The COVID-19 pandemic forces us to reevaluate what is truly important to us as individuals and as a collective. As the tragedy unfolds before us, we are forced to pause and examine our behaviors; we are invited to think of new ways to solve this problem for our own and future generations. May we all persevere and fight for our collective well-being. Despite all the immediate turmoil and peril, life keeps going and the electrophysiology community still needs guidance and education. This issue, finalized during the COVID-19 pandemic, focuses on the treatment of atrial fibrillation (AF), from lifestyle modification to catheter ablation. Specifically, it focuses on different energy sources and balloon approaches to isolate the pulmonary veins. In addition, the issue provides guidance on what to do in patients with recurrent AF and already isolated pulmonary veins and highlights alternative technique and targets for ablation. Extensive narration of non-pulmonary vein triggers approaches is presented. Finally, as atrioesophageal fistula represents the most worrisome complication of AF ablation procedures, techniques for esophageal protection are presented.

Dr Di Biase would like to dedicate this issue to his wife, his future son, his parents, and his family.

Luigi Di Biase, MD, PhD, FACC, FHRS
Albert Einstein College of Medicine
at Montefiore Hospital
Montefiore-Einstein Center for Heart &
Vascular Care
111 East 210th Street
Bronx, NY 10467-2401, USA

Francis Marchlinski, MD, FACC, FHRS
University of Pennsylvania Health System
Hospital of the University of Pennsylvania
Perelman School of Medicine at the University of
Pennsylvania
Philadelphia, PA 19104, USA

Andrea Natale, MD, FACC, FHRS
Texas Cardiac Arrhythmia Institute
Center for Atrial Fibrillation at
St. David's Medical Center
1015 East 32nd Street, Suite 516
Austin, TX 78705, USA

E-mail addresses:
ldibiase@montefiore.org
dibbia@gmail.com (L. Di Biase)
Francis.Marchlinski@pennmedicine.upenn.edu
(F. Marchlinski)
andrea.natale@stdavids.com
Andrea.Natale@stdavidsintl.com (A. Natale)

https://doi.org/10.1016/j.ccep.2020.04.002
1877-9182/20/© 2020 Published by Elsevier Inc.

cardiacEP.theclinics.com

Utility of Cardiac MRI in Atrial Fibrillation Management

Mohammadali Habibi, MD[a], Jonathan Chrispin, MD[a], David D. Spragg, MD[a],
Stefan L. Zimmerman, MD[b], Harikrishna Tandri, MD[a],
Saman Nazarian, MD, PhD[c], Henry Halperin, MD, PhD[a,d],
Natalia Trayanova, PhD[d], Hugh Calkins, MD[a,*]

KEYWORDS

- Cardiac magnetic resonance • Atrial fibrillation • Cardiac MRI

KEY POINTS

- Advances in the cardiac magnetic resonance (CMR) techniques and image acquisition have made it an excellent tool in the assessment of atrial myopathy.
- Remolding of the left atrium (LA), which involves functional, structural, and electrical changes, is the mainstay of atrial fibrillation (AF) development and its progression.
- Given the excellent spatial and temporal resolutions, CMR can detect phasic atrial volumes, atrial function, and atrial fibrosis using cine, and contrast-enhanced or non–contrast-enhanced images.
- These abilities make CMR a versatile and extraordinary tool in management of patients with AF including risk stratification, ablation prognostication and planning, and assessment of stroke risk.

Since the initial application of cardiac magnetic resonance (CMR) in 1980s, it has been increasingly used in structural and functional analysis of the myocardium.[1,2] With improvement in both hardware (eg, coils and higher static field strength) and software (pulse sequence), CMR image acquisition has now become very fast and feasible. In addition, with the growing range of the pulse sequences, it is now possible to perform detailed anatomic, functional, and tissue characterization imaging of the cardiovascular system. Cine images with great spatial resolution and high blood to myocardium and fat to myocardium delineation, and without limitations due to acoustic window, have made CMR the gold standard modality in evaluation of myocardial movement.[3]

Development of gadolinium-based imaging has enabled differentiation of normal and diseased myocardium based on the difference in contrast wash-in and wash-out time.[4,5] Delayed clearance of injected gadolinium from abnormal cardiac tissue leads to enhancement of T1-weighted signals, a phenomenon called late gadolinium enhancement (LGE). In addition, non–contrast-enhanced T1-weighted and T2-weighted (black blood) sequences are another advantage of CMR imaging in detection of acute myocardial injury and edema.[6]

Given the substantial value of CMR, several efforts have been made to enable its utilization in management of patients with atrial fibrillation (AF).[7,8] Many studies suggest the hypothesis of

[a] Division of Cardiology, Section for Cardiac Electrophysiology, Johns Hopkins University, Baltimore, MD, USA; [b] Department of Radiology, Johns Hopkins University, Baltimore, MD, USA; [c] Division of Cardiology, Section for Cardiac Electrophysiology, University of Pennsylvania Perelman School of Medicine, Philadelphia, PA, USA; [d] Department of Biomedical Engineering, Johns Hopkins University, Baltimore, MD, USA
* Corresponding author. Division of Cardiology, The Johns Hopkins Hospital, 1800 Orleans Street, Sheikh Zayed Tower 7125R, Baltimore, MD 21287.
E-mail address: hcalkins@jhmi.edu

Card Electrophysiol Clin 12 (2020) 131–139
https://doi.org/10.1016/j.ccep.2020.02.006
1877-9182/20/© 2020 Elsevier Inc. All rights reserved.

AF as a part atrial myopathy. Therefore, the use of CMR in assessment of atrial myopathy and improvement in management of patients with AF has recently emerged. In this article, we review utilities of CMR in management of patients with AF.

CARDIAC MAGNETIC RESONANCE AND ASSESSMENT OF ATRIAL FIBRILLATION SUBSTRATE

AF is associated with electrical, mechanical, and structural changes in the left atrium (LA).[9] Atrial fibrosis is the hallmark of LA structural changes in patients with AF. Studies have shown that these changes exist before AF development and worsen with AF progression.[10,11] Experimental models have demonstrated that deposition of extracellular matrix and fibrosis create the substrate for promotion and maintenance of AF.[11,12] Gadolinium is a substrate that is not able to cross the intact cell membranes, and therefore, accumulates in the extracellular space. Consequently, atrial fibrotic tissue, which has a higher extracellular volume, retains higher concentration of gadolinium.[11] This results in higher intensity of fibrotic tissue on LGE-CMR compared with healthy myocardium. With advancement of CMR sequences and image resolution, detection and quantification of scar areas within LA have become feasible.[13–15] Relation of fibrotic changes within LA with electrical abnormalities of LA endocardium has been examined in several studies. Spragg and colleagues[16] found a significant association between LGE and areas of low voltage detected by endocardial mapping (Fig. 1). The same findings are also reproduced in other studies with different techniques in quantification of LGE.[17–19] Furthermore, LA LGE is found to be matched with corresponding LA wall areas demonstrating fibrosis on surgical biopsies.[20] The amount of LA LGE is also shown to be higher in patients with persistent AF and more remodeled LA compared with patients with paroxysmal AF.[21]

LA function is another variable that is affected by progression of LA remodeling. LA function can be assessed using both volumetric and deformational analysis methods. Measurement of the volume during the cardiac cycle enables calculation of passive, active, and total LA emptying fraction representatives of conduit, contractile, and global/reservoir functions, respectively.[22] On the other hand, the deformational analysis focuses on the global or regional phasic strain or strain rate. Because of the posterior location and thin wall of the LA, and the complex atrial geometry with presence of pulmonary veins and atrial appendage, accurate assessment of LA function using echocardiography could be challenging. CMR is an excellent tool in assessment of LA volume and function. Feature-tracking CMR can be used not only for measurement of phasic LA volumes, but also is useful in assessment of atrial strain and strain rate with great reproducibility (Fig. 2).[23] Evaluation of LA fibrosis requires optimal sequences and considerable experience in image analysis and variable results have been found depending upon methodologies and institutional experience.[24–26] However, studies using echocardiography and CMR suggest strong associations between the amount of LA fibrosis and worsening LA function.[21,27] In a study by Habibi and colleagues,[21] all phases of LA function were lower in persistent compared with paroxysmal patients with AF and in both compared with healthy volunteers. In this study, the amount of LA LGE was also inversely associated with LA function. CMR assessment of LA volume and function also has a predictive value in AF development. In a case cohort study embedded in the Multi-Ethnic Study of Atherosclerosis (MESA), increased LA volume and lower LA emptying fractions were independent risk factors for incident AF in participants without known cardiovascular disease at baseline.[10] These findings suggest the potential role of CMR in early detection of patients at risk of AF development also as a modality for assessment of LA remodeling progression.

CARDIAC MAGNETIC RESONANCE AND ATRIAL FIBRILLATION ABLATION OUTCOMES

LA LGE has been used in several studies as a marker to prognosticate patients for pulmonary vein isolation (PVI) outcome.[20,28,29] The extent of LA LGE has been categorized by Marrouche and colleagues as stage 1 (<10% of the atrial wall), 2 (≥10% to <20%), 3 (≥20% to <30%), and 4 (≥30%).[28] In the DECAAF (Delayed-Enhancement MRI Determinant of Successful Radiofrequency Catheter Ablation of Atrial Fibrillation) multicenter study in 260 patients who underwent PVI, association of LA fibrosis and recurrent arrhythmia during follow-up was direct and graded (from 15% in stage I group to 51% in the stage IV group).[28] Similar to this study, in a study by Khurram and colleagues[29] in 165 patients with AF, the amount of LA LGE measured with image intensity ratio was associated with recurrent AF. In this study, participants with a low amount of LGE had favorable outcomes regardless of AF persistence at baseline.

In addition to LA LGE, pre-procedural assessment of LA function with CMR has been used successfully to risk stratify patients for AF recurrence after ablation.[30–32] In these studies, LA function

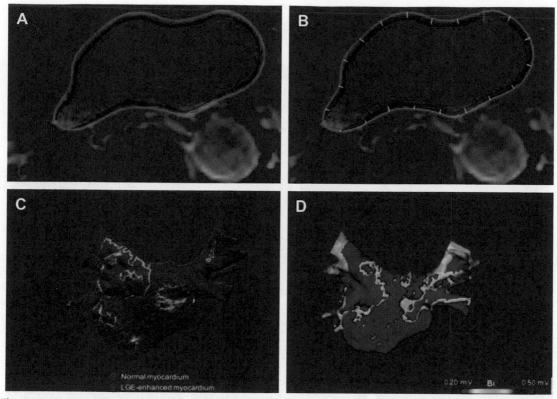

Fig. 1. Assessment of LA fibrosis using CMR LGE. (*A*) A cross section of left atrium with endocardial and epicardial contours. (*B*) Areas of fibrosis based on image intensity ratio are highlighted. (*C*) Shell of left atrial scar areas. (*D*) Endocardial voltage map of left atrium. Comparison of areas with LGE and scar shows excellent correlation.

appears to be superior to LA volume in assessment of LA remodeling and therefore prediction of AF recurrence following ablation. In a study by Dodson and colleagues[31] in 346 patients with AF undergoing PVI, lower passive LA emptying fraction measured during preablation CMR was associated with higher recurrence rate during a 27-month follow-up period. In a study by Habibi and colleagues[30] in 121 patients with paroxysmal and persistent AF, lower baseline LA strain, strain rate, and total LA emptying function measured with feature-tracking CMR were associated with higher AF recurrence during follow-up. This association was independent of known AF risk factors and LA fibrosis measured with LGE-CMR. Atrial dyssynchrony, defined as the standard deviation of the time to the peak longitudinal strain in different atrial segments, is another variable of atrial remodeling that can be measured using feature-tracking CMR. In a study in 208 patients with AF, baseline intra-atrial dyssynchrony during sinus rhythm was an independent predictor of AF recurrence after catheter ablation.[33] Due to asymmetric patterns of LA dilatation, sphericity of LA also has been the subject of studies focusing on

LA remodeling. LA sphericity index, which can be measured using 3-dimensional CMR, compares the variation between actual shape of LA and a sphere (eg, a sphericity index of 1 means that the LA is a perfect sphere).[34] There are few studies showing higher recurrence rate after AF ablation in patients with higher LA sphericity index (more spherical LA remodeling).[34–36]

CARDIAC MAGNETIC RESONANCE TO GUIDE ATRIAL FIBRILLATION ABLATION

Pre-procedural CMR imaging has been used as a guide in AF ablation. Recent evidence suggests that in patients with persistent AF, atrial remodeling and fibrotic changes are the main substrate for susceptibility to AF rather than pulmonary vein triggers. In these patients, atrial fibrosis plays a potential role as an anchor for reentrant arrhythmia circuits.[37,38] Although in a study by Chrispin and colleagues[39] on 9 patients with persistent AF, no association was found between atrial LGE and AF rotors, in another study LGE areas and its amount were linked with locations and the number of regions exhibiting reentrant

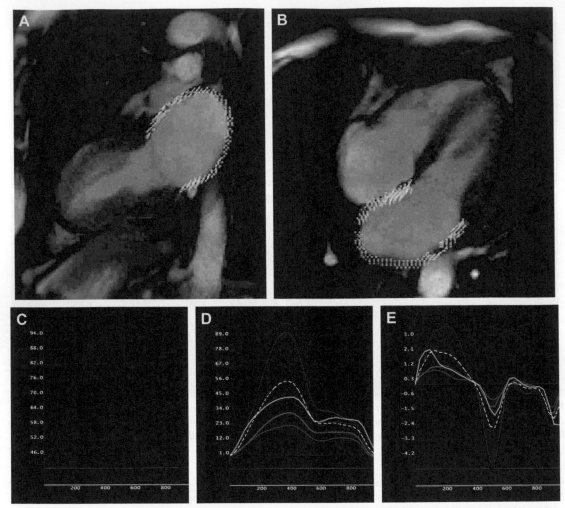

Fig. 2. Feature-tracking CMR and assessment of LA function. Tracking of left atrial myocardium using (*A*) 2-chamber and (*B*) 4-chamber cine images of LA. (*C*) Changes of LA volume during cardiac cycle. (*D*) Segmental LA strain curves. (*E*) Segmental LA strain rate curves.

atrial activity.[40] In addition to reentrant activity, increased LA LGE is also associated with lower local conduction velocity.[41] These findings may explain the suboptimal outcomes of a PVI-alone approach in maintaining sinus rhythm in persistent or long-standing patients with persistent AF who in general have a higher amount of atrial remodeling and LGE.[12] Analysis of CMR images of patients from the DECAAF study reveals that in addition to preablation LGE, residual nonablated atrial fibrosis is also associated with poor outcomes.[42] Therefore, an approach of ablating areas of LGE detected by preablation CMR in addition to PVI may potentially eliminate the substrate and triggers required for initiation and maintenance of AF in patients with nonparoxysmal AF. Outcomes of this approach are being studied in the ongoing DECAAF II trial (NCT02529319). Within the same

concepts, a more personalized approach of using computational atrial modeling using LGE-CMR has been proposed.[43–45] It this approach, a personalized 3-dimensional atrial geometric model is created from segmented pre-procedural CMR images with incorporation of fibrotic and nonfibrotic tissues. Then, region-specific electrical properties are added to the geometric model. Based on the behavior of the model in response to the virtual pacing and predicted locations of reentrant circuits, optimal sets of ablations to fully eliminate the arrhythmogenic property of the substrate is suggested. Boyle and colleagues[46] presented data on feasibility of optimal target identification via modeling of arrhythmogenesis (OPTIMA) in a recent proof of concept study on 10 patients with persistent AF undergoing catheter ablation (**Fig. 3**). If successful in clinical trials, this

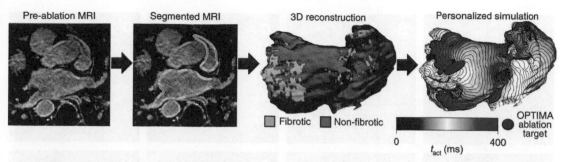

Pre-ablation MRI Segmented MRI 3D reconstruction Personalized simulation

■ Fibrotic ■ Non-fibrotic

OPTIMA ablation target

0 400

t_{act} (ms)

Fig. 3. Algorithm used in the OPTIMA study. LGE mages are used to create a personalized 3-dimensional (3D) atrial model. Then region-specific electrical properties are added to the model. Optimal areas of ablations are proposed based on the behavior of the model in response to virtual pacing.

approach can help improving outcomes of catheter ablation in patients with persistent AF while making the ablation procedure more precise and less time-consuming.

Most cases of AF recurrence after PVI are associated with areas of incomplete ablation or gaps around the pulmonary veins that are not detected during the procedure because of reversible injury and transient conduction block.[47,48] Potential utility of CMR in imaging of acute tissue necrosis and identification of ablation gaps have been investigated in several studies. Acute myocardial lesions can be successfully assessed using either LGE[13,15,49] or noncontrast CMR imaging with T1-weighted[50,51] or T2-weighted pulse sequences.[49,51–54] Although both contrast-enhanced and non–contrast-enhanced CMR can identify acute post ablation lesions, the latter has the advantage of differentiating between permanent ablation lesions from acute transient tissue injury.[55,56] Noncontrast T2-weighted imaging has the ability to enhance the sites of acute ablation; however, it is sensitive to edema, which may lead to overestimation of ablation size.[49,50] In a recent study, Guttman and colleagues[50] proposed a noncontrast T1-weighted sequence with long inversion time that allows a robust visualization of ablation lesions. This sequence was successfully tested in 15 swine with ability to detect permanent radiofrequency ablation lesions in pulmonary vein ostia with good correlations to gross pathology (**Fig. 4**).[57] Preclinical findings of real-time CMR-guided catheter ablation are promising.[58] However, outcomes of real-time CMR-guided AF catheter ablation using noncontrast imaging to guide permanent lesion achievement requires future studies.

Controversial results reported on the ability of LGE-CMR in identification of ablation gaps in patients undergoing a repeat ablation. In a study on 10 patients undergoing repeat ablation, no association was found between scar gaps in CMR and

PV reconnection sites during electroanatomic mapping.[16] However, in another study in 15 patients undergoing repeat AF ablation, the sites of electrical PV reconnection matched with a CMR gap in 79% of PVs.[59] In addition, a CMR-guided approach in targeting the gaps during the repeated ablation resulted in re-isolation of 97% of the reconnected PVs.[59] Relative gap length calculated as the absolute gap length divided by total length of the ablation line measured during CMR at 3 months of follow-up was another marker predicting AF recurrence 1 year after PVI.[60] CMR has been also used successfully for detection of critical isthmus of atrial tachyarrhythmias during a repeat ablation procedure. In this study, CMR scar-based ablation had similar outcomes to electroanatomical mapping guided ablation.[61]

CARDIAC MAGNETIC RESONANCE AND ASSESSMENT FOR RISK OF STROKE

Multiple studies have shown that the extent of atrial remodeling is associated with increased risk of stroke in patients with AF or even in the absence of known AF. Several markers of atrial remodeling such as increase in atrial size[62,63] and changes in P-wave morphology[64] have linked to cerebrovascular events. In most of these studies, the common hypothesis connecting LA structural changes and stroke is the possible role of the assumed LA mechanical or endothelial dysfunction in blood stasis and therefore thromboembolism. In a study by Habibi and colleagues[65] on 4261 individuals without known cardiovascular disease and AF, decreased LA emptying fraction measured with CMR was a predictor of incident ischemic stroke independent of interim incident AF. In other studies in patients with AF, higher atrial LGE,[66,67] decreased LA strain,[68,69] and atrial desynchrony[70] have been predictors of stroke. The amount of LA LGE is also a risk factor for spontaneous echo contrast and atrial appendage

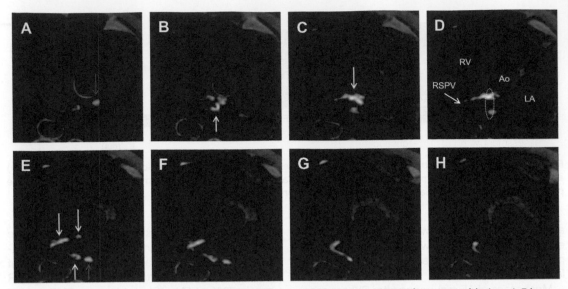

Fig. 4. Non–contrast-enhanced T1-weighted (TWILITE) imaging acutely post radiofrequency ablation. A-E images are horizontal sections through right superior pulmonary vein (RSPV) in cranial to caudal direction. Two locations were ablated in the LA (*orange arrows*) and several around the right superior pulmonary vein ostium (eg, *yellow arrows* in B, C, and E). Lesion enhancement is readily discernible from normal tissue and dark blood. (*D*) The right superior pulmonary vein ostium location is indicated by a dashed yellow ellipse.

thrombus visualized during transesophageal echocardiography.[71] In a study by King and colleagues[67] in 1228 patients with AF, a Utah stage IV versus stage I LA LGE was associated with a fourfold increase risk of previous cerebrovascular events. CMR assessed enlarged left atrial appendage (LAA), and certain LAA characteristics such as extensive trabeculation or certain LAA morphologies also have been associated with increased stroke risk.[72–74] Based on computed tomography and CMR images, Di Biase and colleagues[72] classified LAA morphology as Chicken Wing, Windsock, Cactus, and Cauliflower. The investigators reported that patients with Chicken Wing morphology were less likely to have a history of embolic events.[72] In a study by Khurram and colleagues,[73] LAA orifice size and trabeculation, but not LAA morphology, were associated with higher risk of ischemic stroke.

Currently, risk scores using Congestive Heart Failure, Hypertension, Age, Diabetes, Stroke/Transient Ischemic Attack (CHADS$_2$), or Congestive Heart Failure, Hypertension, Age ($\geq$75 years), Diabetes, Stroke/Transient Ischemic Attack, Vascular Disease, Age (65–74 years), female Sex (CHA$_2$ DS$_2$-VASc) are commonly used in assessment of the risk of stroke and anticoagulation recommendations.[8] Increasing evidence suggests improvement in risk stratification of patients with AF for ischemic stroke by addition of LA remodeling variables to CHADS$_2$ or CHA$_2$ DS$_2$-VASc score.[65,68–70] Outcomes of incorporating atrial

remodeling markers in risk stratification of patients with AF for stroke and decision making on starting anticoagulation needs future studies.

In summary, CMR is an extraordinary versatile technique that yields information on atrial structure, function, tissue characteristics, and blood flow with excellent spatial resolution. Recent studies support the hypothesis that defines AF as a part of LA myopathy. CMR has the potential of revolutionizing the approach to AF management and assessment of LA myopathy. CMR has potential applications in preclinical stage by early detection of LA myopathy. It also can be used in management of patients with AF in preablation prognostication, and planning of ablation strategies. Interventional CMR guiding AF ablation will provide an intriguing window to the personalized medicine end of the atrial imaging spectrum. And finally, CMR can be used in assessment of stroke risk and, therefore, potentially can be incorporated in decision making about anticoagulation planning.

REFERENCES

1. Goldman MR, Brady TJ, Pykett IL, et al. Quantification of experimental myocardial infarction using nuclear magnetic resonance imaging and paramagnetic ion contrast enhancement in excised canine hearts. Circulation 1982;66:1012–6.
2. Herfkens RJ, Higgins CB, Hricak H, et al. Nuclear magnetic resonance imaging of the cardiovascular

system: normal and pathologic findings. Radiology 1983;147:749–59.

3. Foo TK, Bernstein MA, Aisen AM, et al. Improved ejection fraction and flow velocity estimates with use of view sharing and uniform repetition time excitation with fast cardiac techniques. Radiology 1995; 195:471–8.

4. de Roos A, Matheijssen NA, Doornbos J, et al. Myocardial infarct size after reperfusion therapy: assessment with Gd-DTPA-enhanced MR imaging. Radiology 1990;176:517–21.

5. Kim RJ, Wu E, Rafael A, et al. The use of contrast-enhanced magnetic resonance imaging to identify reversible myocardial dysfunction. N Engl J Med 2000;343:1445–53.

6. Simonetti OP, Finn JP, White RD, et al. Black blood" T2-weighted inversion-recovery MR imaging of the heart. Radiology 1996;199:49–57.

7. Calkins H, Willems S, Gerstenfeld EP, et al. Uninterrupted dabigatran versus warfarin for ablation in atrial fibrillation. N Engl J Med 2017;376:1627–36.

8. January CT, Wann LS, Alpert JS, et al. 2014 AHA/ACC/HRS guideline for the management of patients with atrial fibrillation: executive summary: a report of the American College of Cardiology/American Heart Association Task Force on practice guidelines and the Heart Rhythm Society. Circulation 2014;130: 2071–104.

9. Allessie M, Ausma J, Schotten U. Electrical, contractile and structural remodeling during atrial fibrillation. Cardiovasc Res 2002;54:230–46.

10. Habibi M, Samiei S, Ambale Venkatesh B, et al. Cardiac magnetic resonance-measured left atrial volume and function and incident atrial fibrillation: results from MESA (Multi-Ethnic Study of Atherosclerosis). Circ Cardiovasc Imaging 2016;9 [pii: e004299].

11. Burstein B, Nattel S. Atrial fibrosis: mechanisms and clinical relevance in atrial fibrillation. J Am Coll Cardiol 2008;51:802–9.

12. Delgado V, Di Biase L, Leung M, et al. Structure and function of the left atrium and left atrial appendage: AF and stroke implications. J Am Coll Cardiol 2017; 70:3157–72.

13. Peters DC, Wylie JV, Hauser TH, et al. Detection of pulmonary vein and left atrial scar after catheter ablation with three-dimensional navigator-gated delayed enhancement MR imaging: initial experience. Radiology 2007;243:690–5.

14. Oakes RS, Badger TJ, Kholmovski EG, et al. Detection and quantification of left atrial structural remodeling with delayed-enhancement magnetic resonance imaging in patients with atrial fibrillation. Circulation 2009;119:1758–67.

15. McGann CJ, Kholmovski EG, Oakes RS, et al. New magnetic resonance imaging-based method for defining the extent of left atrial wall injury after the ablation of atrial fibrillation. J Am Coll Cardiol 2008; 52:1263–71.

16. Spragg DD, Khurram I, Zimmerman SL, et al. Initial experience with magnetic resonance imaging of atrial scar and co-registration with electroanatomic voltage mapping during atrial fibrillation: success and limitations. Heart Rhythm 2012;9:2003–9.

17. Jadidi AS, Cochet H, Shah AJ, et al. Inverse relationship between fractionated electrograms and atrial fibrosis in persistent atrial fibrillation: combined magnetic resonance imaging and high-density mapping. J Am Coll Cardiol 2013;62:802–12.

18. Khurram IM, Beinart R, Zipunnikov V, et al. Magnetic resonance image intensity ratio, a normalized measure to enable interpatient comparability of left atrial fibrosis. Heart Rhythm 2014;11:85–92.

19. Malcolme-Lawes LC, Juli C, Karim R, et al. Automated analysis of atrial late gadolinium enhancement imaging that correlates with endocardial voltage and clinical outcomes: a 2-center study. Heart Rhythm 2013;10:1184–91.

20. McGann C, Akoum N, Patel A, et al. Atrial fibrillation ablation outcome is predicted by left atrial remodeling on MRI. Circ Arrhythm Electrophysiol 2014;7: 23–30.

21. Habibi M, Lima JA, Khurram IM, et al. Association of left atrial function and left atrial enhancement in patients with atrial fibrillation: cardiac magnetic resonance study. Circ Cardiovasc Imaging 2015;8: e002769.

22. Hoit BD. Left atrial size and function: role in prognosis. J Am Coll Cardiol 2014;63(6):493–505.

23. Zareian M, Ciuffo L, Habibi M, et al. Left atrial structure and functional quantitation using cardiovascular magnetic resonance and multimodality tissue tracking: validation and reproducibility assessment. J Cardiovasc Magn Reson 2015;17:52.

24. Chrispin J, Ipek EG, Habibi M, et al. Clinical predictors of cardiac magnetic resonance late gadolinium enhancement in patients with atrial fibrillation. Europace 2017;19:371–7.

25. Mahnkopf C, Badger TJ, Burgon NS, et al. Evaluation of the left atrial substrate in patients with lone atrial fibrillation using delayed-enhanced MRI: implications for disease progression and response to catheter ablation. Heart rhythm 2010;7:1475–81.

26. Siebermair J, Suksaranjit P, McGann CJ, et al. Atrial fibrosis in non-atrial fibrillation individuals and prediction of atrial fibrillation by use of late gadolinium enhancement magnetic resonance imaging. J Cardiovasc Electrophysiol 2019;30:550–6.

27. Kuppahally SS, Akoum N, Burgon NS, et al. Left atrial strain and strain rate in patients with paroxysmal and persistent atrial fibrillation: relationship to left atrial structural remodeling detected by delayed-enhancement MRI. Circ Cardiovasc Imaging 2010;3:231–9.

28. Marrouche NF, Wilber D, Hindricks G, et al. Association of atrial tissue fibrosis identified by delayed enhancement MRI and atrial fibrillation catheter ablation: the DECAAF study. JAMA 2014;311:498–506.

29. Khurram IM, Habibi M, Gucuk Ipek E, et al. Left atrial LGE and arrhythmia recurrence following pulmonary vein isolation for paroxysmal and persistent AF. JACC Cardiovasc Imaging 2016;9:142–8.

30. Habibi M, Lima JA, Gucuk Ipek E, et al. The association of baseline left atrial structure and function measured with cardiac magnetic resonance and pulmonary vein isolation outcome in patients with drug-refractory atrial fibrillation. Heart rhythm 2016;13:1037–44.

31. Dodson JA, Neilan TG, Shah RV, et al. Left atrial passive emptying function determined by cardiac magnetic resonance predicts atrial fibrillation recurrence after pulmonary vein isolation. Circ Cardiovasc Imaging 2014;7:586–92.

32. Chubb H, Karim R, Mukherjee R, et al. A comprehensive multi-index cardiac magnetic resonance-guided assessment of atrial fibrillation substrate prior to ablation: prediction of long-term outcomes. J Cardiovasc Electrophysiol 2019;30:1894–903.

33. Ciuffo L, Tao S, Gucuk Ipek E, et al. Intra-atrial dyssynchrony during sinus rhythm predicts recurrence after the first catheter ablation for atrial fibrillation. JACC Cardiovasc Imaging 2019;12:310–9.

34. Bisbal F, Guiu E, Calvo N, et al. Left atrial sphericity: a new method to assess atrial remodeling. impact on the outcome of atrial fibrillation ablation. J Cardiovasc Electrophysiol 2013;24:752–9.

35. Bisbal F, Alarcon F, Ferrero-de-Loma-Osorio A, et al. Left atrial geometry and outcome of atrial fibrillation ablation: results from the multicentre LAGO-AF study. Eur Heart J Cardiovasc Imaging 2018;19:1002–9.

36. Moon J, Lee HJ, Yu J, et al. Prognostic implication of left atrial sphericity in atrial fibrillation patients undergoing radiofrequency catheter ablation. Pacing Clin Electrophysiol 2017;40:713–20.

37. Ashihara T, Haraguchi R, Nakazawa K, et al. The role of fibroblasts in complex fractionated electrograms during persistent/permanent atrial fibrillation: implications for electrogram-based catheter ablation. Circ Res 2012;110:275–84.

38. Gonzales MJ, Vincent KP, Rappel WJ, et al. Structural contributions to fibrillatory rotors in a patient-derived computational model of the atria. Europace 2014;16(Suppl 4):iv3–10.

39. Chrispin J, Gucuk Ipek E, Zahid S, et al. Lack of regional association between atrial late gadolinium enhancement on cardiac magnetic resonance and atrial fibrillation rotors. Heart rhythm 2016;13:654–60.

40. Cochet H, Dubois R, Yamashita S, et al. Relationship between fibrosis detected on late gadolinium-enhanced cardiac magnetic resonance and re-entrant activity assessed with electrocardiographic imaging in human persistent atrial fibrillation. JACC Clin Electrophysiol 2018;4:17–29.

41. Fukumoto K, Habibi M, Ipek EG, et al. Association of left atrial local conduction velocity with late gadolinium enhancement on cardiac magnetic resonance in patients with atrial fibrillation. Circ Arrhythm Electrophysiol 2016;9:e002897.

42. Akoum N, Wilber D, Hindricks G, et al. MRI assessment of ablation-induced scarring in atrial fibrillation: analysis from the DECAAF Study. J Cardiovasc Electrophysiol 2015;26:473–80.

43. McDowell KS, Zahid S, Vadakkumpadan F, et al. Virtual electrophysiological study of atrial fibrillation in fibrotic remodeling. PLoS One 2015;10:e0117110.

44. Roney CH, Bayer JD, Zahid S, et al. Modelling methodology of atrial fibrosis affects rotor dynamics and electrograms. Europace 2016;18:iv146–55.

45. Zahid S, Cochet H, Boyle PM, et al. Patient-derived models link re-entrant driver localization in atrial fibrillation to fibrosis spatial pattern. Cardiovasc Res 2016;110:443–54.

46. Boyle PM, Zghaib T, Zahid S, et al. Computationally guided personalized targeted ablation of persistent atrial fibrillation. Nat Biomed Eng 2019;3(11):870–9.

47. Ouyang F, Antz M, Ernst S, et al. Recovered pulmonary vein conduction as a dominant factor for recurrent atrial tachyarrhythmias after complete circular isolation of the pulmonary veins: lessons from double Lasso technique. Circulation 2005;111:127–35.

48. Wood MA, Fuller IA. Acute and chronic electrophysiologic changes surrounding radiofrequency lesions. J Cardiovasc Electrophysiol 2002;13:56–61.

49. Dickfeld T, Kato R, Zviman M, et al. Characterization of radiofrequency ablation lesions with gadolinium-enhanced cardiovascular magnetic resonance imaging. J Am Coll Cardiol 2006;47:370–8.

50. Guttman MA, Tao S, Fink S, et al. Non-contrast-enhanced T1 -weighted MRI of myocardial radiofrequency ablation lesions. Magn Reson Med 2018;79:879–89.

51. Lardo AC, McVeigh ER, Jumrussirikul P, et al. Visualization and temporal/spatial characterization of cardiac radiofrequency ablation lesions using magnetic resonance imaging. Circulation 2000;102:698–705.

52. Zghaib T, Malayeri AA, Ipek EG, et al. Visualization of acute edema in the left atrial myocardium after radiofrequency ablation: application of a novel high-resolution 3-dimensional magnetic resonance imaging sequence. Heart rhythm 2018;15:1189–97.

53. Chubb H, Harrison JL, Weiss S, et al. Development, preclinical validation, and clinical translation of a cardiac magnetic resonance - electrophysiology

system with active catheter tracking for ablation of cardiac arrhythmia. JACC Clin Electrophysiol 2017; 3:89–103.

54. Vergara GR, Vijayakumar S, Kholmovski EG, et al. Real-time magnetic resonance imaging-guided radiofrequency atrial ablation and visualization of lesion formation at 3 Tesla. Heart rhythm 2011;8: 295–303.

55. Dall'Armellina E, Karia N, Lindsay AC, et al. Dynamic changes of edema and late gadolinium enhancement after acute myocardial infarction and their relationship to functional recovery and salvage index. Circ Cardiovasc Imaging 2011;4:228–36.

56. Ghafoori E, Kholmovski EG, Thomas S, et al. Characterization of gadolinium contrast enhancement of radiofrequency ablation lesions in predicting edema and chronic lesion size. Circ Arrhythm Electrophysiol 2017;10 [pii:e005599].

57. Guttman MA, Tao S, Fink S, et al. Acute enhancement of necrotic radio-frequency ablation lesions in left atrium and pulmonary vein ostia in swine model with non-contrast-enhanced T1-weighted MRI. Magn Reson Med 2020;83(4):1368–79.

58. Piorkowski C, Grothoff M, Gaspar T, et al. Cavotricuspid isthmus ablation guided by real-time magnetic resonance imaging. Circ Arrhythm Electrophysiol 2013;6:e7–10.

59. Bisbal F, Guiu E, Cabanas-Grandio P, et al. CMR-guided approach to localize and ablate gaps in repeat AF ablation procedure. JACC Cardiovasc Imaging 2014;7:653–63.

60. Linhart M, Alarcon F, Borras R, et al. Delayed gadolinium enhancement magnetic resonance imaging detected anatomic gap length in wide circumferential pulmonary vein ablation lesions is associated with recurrence of atrial fibrillation. Circ Arrhythm Electrophysiol 2018;11:e006659.

61. Fochler F, Yamaguchi T, Kheirkhan M, et al. Late gadolinium enhancement magnetic resonance imaging guided treatment of post-atrial fibrillation ablation recurrent arrhythmia. Circ Arrhythm Electrophysiol 2019;12:e007174.

62. Benjamin EJ, D'Agostino RB, Belanger AJ, et al. Left atrial size and the risk of stroke and death. The Framingham Heart Study. Circulation 1995;92:835–41.

63. Di Tullio MR, Sacco RL, Sciacca RR, et al. Left atrial size and the risk of ischemic stroke in an ethnically mixed population. Stroke 1999;30:2019–24.

64. Kamel H, O'Neal WT, Okin PM, et al. Electrocardiographic left atrial abnormality and stroke subtype in the atherosclerosis risk in communities study. Ann Neurol 2015;78:670–8.

65. Habibi M, Zareian M, Ambale Venkatesh B, et al. Left atrial mechanical function and incident ischemic cerebrovascular events independent of AF: insights from the MESA study. JACC Cardiovasc Imaging 2019;12(12):2417–27.

66. Daccarett M, Badger TJ, Akoum N, et al. Association of left atrial fibrosis detected by delayed-enhancement magnetic resonance imaging and the risk of stroke in patients with atrial fibrillation. J Am Coll Cardiol 2011;57:831–8.

67. King JB, Azadani PN, Suksaranjit P, et al. Left atrial fibrosis and risk of cerebrovascular and cardiovascular events in patients with atrial fibrillation. J Am Coll Cardiol 2017;70:1311–21.

68. Inoue YY, Alissa A, Khurram IM, et al. Quantitative tissue-tracking cardiac magnetic resonance (CMR) of left atrial deformation and the risk of stroke in patients with atrial fibrillation. J Am Heart Assoc 2015;4 [pii:e001844].

69. Azemi T, Rabdiya VM, Ayirala SR, et al. Left atrial strain is reduced in patients with atrial fibrillation, stroke or TIA, and low risk CHADS(2) scores. J Am Soc Echocardiogr 2012;25:1327–32.

70. Ciuffo L, Inoue YY, Tao S, et al. Mechanical dyssynchrony of the left atrium during sinus rhythm is associated with history of stroke in patients with atrial fibrillation. Eur Heart J Cardiovasc Imaging 2018; 19:433–41.

71. Akoum N, Fernandez G, Wilson B, et al. Association of atrial fibrosis quantified using LGE-MRI with atrial appendage thrombus and spontaneous contrast on transesophageal echocardiography in patients with atrial fibrillation. J Cardiovasc Electrophysiol 2013; 24:1104–9.

72. Di Biase L, Santangeli P, Anselmino M, et al. Does the left atrial appendage morphology correlate with the risk of stroke in patients with atrial fibrillation? Results from a multicenter study. J Am Coll Cardiol 2012;60:531–8.

73. Khurram IM, Dewire J, Mager M, et al. Relationship between left atrial appendage morphology and stroke in patients with atrial fibrillation. Heart rhythm 2013;10:1843–9.

74. Beinart R, Heist EK, Newell JB, et al. Left atrial appendage dimensions predict the risk of stroke/TIA in patients with atrial fibrillation. J Cardiovasc Electrophysiol 2011;22:10–5.

Risk Factor Management Before and After Atrial Fibrillation Ablation

Jonathan P. Ariyaratnam, MB BChir[a], Melissa Middeldorp, PhD[a],
Gijo Thomas, PhD[b], Jean Jacques Noubiap, MD[a], Dennis Lau, MBBS, PhD[a],
Prashanthan Sanders, MBBS, PhD[a],*

KEYWORDS

- Atrial fibrillation • Catheter ablation • Risk factor management

KEY POINTS

- Modifiable risk factors including hypertension, diabetes, obesity, sleep apnea, alcohol consumption, physical inactivity and smoking have a pivotal role in the development and progression of atrial fibrillation.
- Risk factor management is critical to optimizing management of atrial fibrillation.
- Outcomes of catheter ablation of atrial fibrillation are significantly improved through aggressive monitoring and treatment of risk factors both before and after ablation.
- Risk factor management programs are cost-effective interventions with the ability to effectively educate and motivate patients to improve lifestyle and better control modifiable risk factors.

INTRODUCTION

Atrial fibrillation (AF) continues to be associated with significant all-cause mortality risk and increasing health care cost burden. Hospitalizations due to AF have now overtaken those of myocardial infarction and heart failure demonstrating the increasing need for improved treatments.[1] Currently, AF ablation remains the optimum method for rhythm control, with long-term efficacy rates after multiple procedures reaching 80% for paroxysmal AF.[2] AF ablation efficacy continues to be associated, however, with significant attrition over time.[3–6] Reduction in these attrition rates represents a potential target for improving outcomes associated with AF.

Risk factor management (RFM) is an essential pillar of care for AF management with evidence suggesting that it can reduce attrition associated with AF ablation.[7] RFM involves the aggressive identification, monitoring, and treatment of important cardiovascular risk factors, such as hypertension, diabetes, obesity, sleep apnea, and physical inactivity. Current clinical guidelines for the management of AF strongly advocate RFM based on several recent studies showing that RFM improves patients' symptoms, quality of life, and long-term outcomes.[7–10] Although interventional AF ablation continues to play an important part in the overall strategy for management of AF, aggressive RFM optimizes patients preprocedurally and maximizes and prolongs the benefits postprocedurally.

MODIFIABLE RISK FACTORS ASSOCIATED WITH ATRIAL FIBRILLATION

Several modifiable risk factors have been identified as important independent risk factors for the development of AF. These risk factors are thought to induce hemodynamic and/or electrophysiologic

[a] Centre for Heart Rhythm Disorders, University of Adelaide, Royal Adelaide Hospital, Adelaide, South Australia 5000, Australia; [b] Centre for Heart Rhythm Disorders, University of Adelaide, South Australian Health and Medical Research Institute (SAHMRI) Adelaide, SA 5000, Australia
* Corresponding author. Director, Centre for Heart Rhythm Disorders, University of Adelaide and Royal Adelaide Hospital, Adelaide, SA 5000, Australia.
E-mail address: prash.sanders@adelaide.edu.au

Card Electrophysiol Clin 12 (2020) 141–154
https://doi.org/10.1016/j.ccep.2020.02.009
1877-9182/20/Crown Copyright © 2020 Published by Elsevier Inc. All rights reserved.

Table 1
Independent risk of incident AF according to presence of individual risk factors

Risk Factor	Study	Study Type	Number of Patients	Definition	Follow-up (y)	Risk Estimate for incident AF (95% confidence interval
Hypertension	Framingham Heart Study,[11] 1994	Observational cohort	1948	Systolic >160 mm Hg OR diastolic >95 mm Hg	38	Male: 1.5 (1.2–2.0) Female: 1.4 (1.1–1.8)
	ARIC study,[59] 2011	Observational cohort	4852 1648	Systolic BP 120–<140 Systolic BP 140–<160	10	1.42 (1.15–1.76) 2.16 (1.67–2.79)
Diabetes	Aune et al,[16] 2018	Meta-analysis	10,244, 043	Any diagnosis diabetes mellitus	>10	1.37 (1.25–1.5)
Obesity	Asad et al,[60] 2018	Meta-analysis	587,372	BMI >30 kg/m^2	13.6	1.51 (1.365–1.68)
Obstructive sleep apnea	Youssef et al,[25] 2018	Meta-analysis	19,837	AHI >5 3% ODI >15 events RDI >30 events	Not recorded	2.12 (1.845–2.436)
Alcohol consumption	Gallagher et al,[29] 2017	Meta-analysis	249,496	3 or more standard drinks (10–12 g)/d	4–17.6	1.4 (1.19–1.64)
Smoking	Aune et al,[61] 2018	Meta-analysis	388,030	Current smokers vs never smokers	Not recorded	1.32 (1.12–1.56)
Physical inactivity	Mohanty et al,[38] 2016	Meta-analysis	93,995	Sedentary vs nonsedentary	6	2.47 (1.25–3.6)

Large studies showing that the presence of hypertension, diabetes, obesity, sleep apnea, alcohol consumption, cigarette smoking, and physical inactivity each independently and significantly increase the risk of incident AF. AF, atrial fibrillation; AHI, apnea-hypopnea index; ARIC, atherosclerosis risk in communities; BMI, body mass index; RDI, respiratory disturbance index; ODI, oxygen desaturation index.

changes within the left atrium, creating the milieu for AF development. **Table 1** identifies studies showing the independent effect of each cardiovascular risk factor on the risk of development of AF.

Hypertension

Hypertension is a key cardiovascular risk factor known to be strongly associated with AF. In the Framingham Heart Study, people were 40% to 50% more likely to develop AF if they were hypertensive.[11] Furthermore, treatment of hypertension, targeting a systolic blood pressure (BP) of less than 130 mm Hg, has been shown to reduce the risk of incident AF by up to 40%.[12] Hypertension, therefore, has been shown to be a key modifiable risk factor for the development of new AF.

The basic mechanisms underlying this important association are related to left atrial structural and electrophysiologic remodeling. Systemic hypertension results in increased afterload and, therefore, pressure overload on the left ventricle. To compensate, the left ventricle hypertrophies and stiffens, leading to reduced diastolic left ventricular filling and increased volume within the left atrium. The left atrium subsequently dilates resulting in the electrophysiologic changes associated with AF. In addition, the increased circulating levels of angiotensin II released by the renal system in hypertension have a direct effect on the cells of the atria, resulting in atrial fibrosis and electrophysiologic remodeling.[13–15]

Diabetes

Several studies have confirmed diabetes mellitus (both type 1 and type 2) as an independent risk factor for incident AF, increasing the risk by 37%.[16] Through increased production of reactive oxygen species and advanced glycation end products, diabetes has been shown to result in fibrotic change as well as ion channel and gap junction remodeling within the atria.[17,18] These changes increase conduction heterogeneity, reduce conduction velocity, and prolong the action potential, creating the electrophysiologic conditions for the development of AF.

Obesity

Obesity is global epidemic and a major driver of the increasing prevalence of AF worldwide. Every 5-point increment in body mass index (BMI) has been shown to independently increase the risk of AF by 29%.[19] Mechanisms again include structural and electrophysiological remodelling of the atria through alterations in cardiovascular haemodynamics as well as fibrotic and ion channel remodelling.[20–22] In addition, cardiac imaging studies have shown that obesity is associated with increased epicardial and pericardial fat deposition adjacent to the left atrium.[23] Increased pericardial and epicardial fat is associated with AF, likely through direct fatty infiltration of the left atrium in addition to paracrine effects attributable to released cytokines and chemokines.[24]

Obstructive Sleep Apnea

Obstructive sleep apnea (OSA) is a chronic condition characterized by recurrent pharyngeal collapse, leading to repetitive interruption of ventilation during sleep. It is increasingly recognized as a critical risk factor in a variety of cardiovascular conditions and recently has been identified as an independent risk factor for incident AF. The presence of sleep apnea doubles the risk of incident AF.[25] Both the acute effects of apneic episodes and the chronic effects of long-term OSA are thought to contribute to the increased risk of AF. The transient hypoxemia associated with pharyngeal collapse is postulated to result in changes in atrial effective refractory periods acutely, resulting in increased susceptibility to induction and maintenance of AF.[26] Additionally, chronic OSA results in significant hemodynamic changes, which increase left atrial pressures, thereby resulting in left atrial enlargement.[27] Chronic OSA also is known to induce a systemic inflammatory and prothrombotic state, which increases the likelihood of fibrotic change and electrophysiologic remodeling within the atria.[28]

Alcohol Consumption

Long-term alcohol intake has been shown to be associated with AF in a dose-dependent manner.[29] High quantities of alcohol consumption (more than 3 standard drinks per day) increase the risk of AF development by approximately 40%, with a more significant effect in men. Proposed mechanisms for this important association include direct effects of alcohol on atrial electrophysiology (conduction slowing and shortening of the atrial effective refractory period),[30] alterations in autonomic nervous control of the heart,[31] and an increase in circulating plasma free fatty acids, which have been shown to be arrhythmogenic.[32] Structural remodeling of the left atrium also may underly the association, with evidence that chronic alcohol consumption leads to left atrial enlargement.[33] Of course, chronic alcohol consumption is closely associated with other independent risk factors, including hypertension, obesity, and sleep apnea.

Smoking

Several long-term prospective observational cohort studies have identified smoking as an independent predictor of incident AF.[34–36] Furthermore, a majority of these studies showed that the risk was higher in those who continued to smoke compared with those who quit smoking. The link between smoking and AF is unsurprising; smoking induces oxidative stress, inflammation, and atrial fibrosis, all of which predispose to AF. In addition, it has been shown that smoking increases risk of thromboembolism and mortality in those with AF, providing strong evidence that smoking cessation should be a critical factor in mitigating AF risk.[37]

Physical Inactivity

Physical activity and exercise are inextricably linked with cardiovascular health. Increasing evidence suggests that sedentary lifestyles increase the risk of incident AF.[38] Regular light-to-moderate exercise has been shown to reduce the risk of the development of AF by up to 28%.[39] The relationship between physical exercise and incident AF, however, does not appear to be linear; a recent large cohort study of more than 500 thousand participants in Korea showed that the relationship was U-shaped, with highly active subjects (>1000 metabolic equivalent of task [MET] minutes/wk) exhibiting increased risk of incident AF compared with moderately active individuals.[40] Regular moderate-intensity exercise, therefore, appears the key in reducing risk of AF.

RISK FACTOR MANAGEMENT IN ATRIAL FIBRILLATION

Given the overwhelming epidemiologic evidence linking these risk factors with incident AF, it is no surprise that there is growing interest in RFM as a treatment modality for management of AF. RFM involves the systematic search for poorly controlled modifiable risk factors and the initiation of treatments (lifestyle, medical, and interventional) in order to better control these risk factors. Specific interventions focusing on risk factors, such as tightly regulated blood pressure and blood sugars, significant weight loss through improved diet and exercise, treatment of OSA with continuous positive airway pressure (CPAP), increased physical activity, alcohol reduction, and smoking cessation, are increasingly linked to improved outcomes associated with AF. Several studies have demonstrated that treatment of individual risk factors as well as all-encompassing comprehensive RFM programs can significantly improve outcomes associated with AF, both before and after ablation.[7,10,41,42,43]

RISK FACTOR MANAGEMENT BEFORE ABLATION

Table 2 presents studies providing evidence for improved AF outcomes associated with various RFM strategies initiated before ablation. The biggest effect has been seen with overarching RFM programmes comprehensively targeting all relevant modifiable risk factors including hypertension, diabetes, OSA, overweight or obesity, physical inactivity, smoking and alcohol consumption.[8–10] More recently, bariatric surgery in a morbidly obese population was shown to result in significant improvements in BMI, blood pressure and blood glucose control and ultimately enhanced sinus rhythm maintenance after AF ablation.[44] Even management of individual risk factors alone, however, has been shown effective in improving AF outcomes; treatment of OSA with CPAP prior to AF ablation has been shown to improve the efficacy of any subsequent AF ablation.[42,45] In addition, the Cardiorespiratory Fitness on Arrhythmia Recurrence in Obese Individuals with Atrial Fibrillation (CARDIO-FIT) study showed that gains in cardiorespiratory fitness were independently associated with significant improvements in AF outcomes,[43] while medical management of hypertension preablation also has been shown effective in improving ablation outcomes.[46] In a more recent study, aggressive treatment of hypertension

leading to a reduction in systolic blood pressure of ~ 20 mmHg resulted in a 42% reduction in risk of recurrent AF after ablation, but this benefit was restricted to older patients (≥ 61 years).[47] In general, studies investigating outcomes after multiple ablation procedures and longer follow-up durations have consistently demonstrated improvements with RFM before ablation.[9,10,41,43]

RISK FACTOR MANAGEMENT AFTER ATRIAL FIBRILLATION ABLATION
Independent Predictors of Atrial Fibrillation Recurrence after Ablation

Very late recurrence of AF even after multiple ablation procedures remains a significant problem in the management of AF. Several predictors for AF recurrence have been proposed, including type of AF, duration of AF, left atrial volume, and ejection fraction.[48] Cardiovascular risk factors, however, also have been shown to be important predictors of AF recurrence after ablation. Table 3 shows pooled risk estimates for recurrence of AF after ablation associated with individual independent risk factors. There is now a large body of evidence to suggest that the aforementioned risk factors are important independent predictors for AF recurrence when present after ablation.

Risk Factor Management Improves Outcomes After Ablation

The fact that risk factors are associated with AF recurrence after ablation suggests that RFM postablation may improve long-term outcomes. Table 4 identifies studies providing evidence for improved AF outcomes associated with RFM strategies initiated after AF ablation. The Aggressive Risk Factor Reduction Study for Atrial Fibrillation and Implications for the Outcome of Ablation (AR-REST-AF) study compared routine postablation care with an aggressive physician-directed RFM program.[7] Patients in the RFM group were reviewed in a specific 3-monthly RFM clinic, where a structured motivational and goal-directed program using face-to-face counseling was used to enable lifestyle modifications. In addition, smoking cessation and alcohol reduction were actively encouraged while pharmacotherapy and CPAP were initiated for treatment of hypertension, diabetes, and sleep apnea. After more than 3 years of follow-up, the RFM group lost significantly more weight and experienced improved control of blood pressure, blood sugars, and sleep apnea in comparison to the control group. The patients in the RFM group went on to experience reduced AF-related symptoms and improved global well-being and were significantly less likely to exhibit

Table 2
Effect of RFM prior to ablation on long-term outcomes of catheter ablation for AF

Study	Type of Study	Preablation Intervention	Population	Changes in Risk Factors	Average Duration of Follow-up (months)	Number of Procedures	Outcomes
Ablation-specific outcomes							
Donnellan et al,[44] 2019	Cohort	Bariatric surgery	239 morbidly obese patients • 51 bariatric surgery • 188 medical management of obesity	Intervention group • Mean systolic BP 144.9–117.8 • Mean BMI 47.6–36.8 kg/m$_2$ • HbA$_{1c}$ 6.7–5.8	36	Multiple	Reduced AF recurrence postablation at 3 y (HR 0.382; 95% CI, 0.167–0.875)
Mohanty et al,[62] 2018	Cohort	Weight loss through dietary and exercise interventions	90 obese patients • 58 weight loss intervention • 32 no weight loss intervention	Median weight loss 24.9 kg	9	Single	No significant difference in ablation outcome ($P = .68$)
Parkash et al,[63] 2017	Randomized clinical trial	Medical management of blood pressure	173 AF patients with BP >130/80 • 88 intervention group • 85 control group	Mean BP at follow-up • Intervention group— 123.2/76.7 • Control group— 135.4/80.8	14	Single	Recurrence risk after ablation in intervention group compared with control group 0.94 (95% CI, 0.65–1.38)
Pathak et al,[9] 2017 (CENT study)	Cohort	Aggressive RFM	355 AF patients with BMI >27 • 208 RFM • 147 no RFM	BP <130/80 mm Hg, 10% weight loss, all risk factors targeted	47.03 (intervention group); 49.01 (controls)	Multiple	Arrythmia-free survival 77% in RFM group compared with 40% in control group ($P<.001$)
Santoro et al,[46] 2015	Cohort	Medical treatment of hypertension	531 participants, 3 groups • 160 uncontrolled hypertension • 192 controlled hypertension	• Uncontrolled hypertension— mean SBP 156.6 • Controlled hypertension— mean SBP 127.7	19	Single	Recurrence risk ablation • Uncontrolled hypertension 1.52 (95% CI, 1.01–2.29)

(continued on next page)

Table 2
(*continued*)

Study	Type of Study	Preablation Intervention	Population	Changes in Risk Factors	Average Duration of Follow-up (months)	Number of Procedures	Outcomes
			• 179 no hypertension				• Controlled hypertension 1.05 (95% CI, 0.70–1.58)
OSA studies 1. Fein et al, 2013[42] 2. Bazan et al, 2013[63] 3. Patel et al, 2010[45] 4. Jongnarangsin et al, 2008[64]	Cohort	CPAP	AF patients with OSA diagnosed on polysomnography	Gold standard treatment of OSA	1. 12 2. 12 3. 20 4. 7	All single	Overall reduced risk of AF recurrence after ablation 1. 0.44 (0.24–0.82) 2. 1.30 (0.30–2.48) 3. 0.62 (0.46–0.83) 4. 0.70 (0.40–1.24)
Long term arrhythmia-free outcomes (with/without ablation)							
Pathak et al,[10] 2015 (LEGACY)	Prospective observational cohort	Aggressive RFM	355 AF patients with BMI >27 • 135 >10% weight loss (group 1) • 103 3%–10% weight loss (group 2) • <3% weight loss (group 3)	BP <130/80 mm Hg, 10% weight loss, all risk factors targeted	48.4 (group 1); 46.0 (group 2); 48.3 (group 3)	Multiple	Risk of AF recurrence • Group 1–1.00 (reference) • Group 2–3.1 (95% CI, 1.7–5.6) • Group 3–5.9 (95% CI, 3.4–10.9)
Pathak et al,[43] 2015 (CARDIO-FIT)	Prospective observational cohort	Cardiorespiratory fitness gains	308 AF patients with BMI >27 • 127 >2 METs gain • 181 <2 METs gain	Cardiorespiratory fitness gain >2 METs	49	Multiple	Arrythmia-free survival 89% in gain >2 METs group compared with 40% in gain <2 METs group (*P*<.001)

Details of studies investigating the impact of the management (lifestyle, medical, and interventional) of individual and multiple risk factors prior to AF ablation procedure on AF ablation outcomes. AF, atrial fibrillation; BP, blood pressure; BMI, body mass index; CI, confidence interval; CPAP, continuous positive airway pressure; MET, metabolic equivalent of tasks; OSA, obstructive sleep apnea; RFM, risk factor management; SBP, systolic blood pressure.

Table 3
Independent predictors of AF recurrence after catheter ablation for AF

Risk Factor	Number of Studies	Number of Patients	Definition	Pooled Adjusted Risk Estimate (Hazard ratios) for Atrial Fibrillation Recurrence After Atrial Fibrillation Ablation Procedures (95% Confidence interval)
Hypertension	24	11,099	Any diagnosis hypertension	1.40 (1.23–1.59)
Diabetes	11	7954	Any diagnosis diabetes	1.37 (1.19–1.60)
Obesity	9	8662	BMI >30 kg/m$_2$	1.38 (1.15–1.65)
Epicardial fat (Wong et al,[19] 2015)	11	1527	Per 1 SD increase in epicardial fat volume	2.69 (1.66–4.07)
Obstructive sleep apnea	5	4321	AHI >15	1.94 (1.15–3.25)

Pooled independent risk estimates for the recurrence of AF after AF ablation according to the presence of individual risk factors. Studies identifying risk factors as independent predictors of AF recurrence included in the pooled analysis. Hazard ratios and CIs extracted from published studies. Pooled hazard ratios calculated using random-effects model. AF, atrial fibrillation; AHI, apnea-hyponea index; BMI, body mass index; SD, standard deviation.

recurrence of AF after ablation. Additionally, renal artery denervation has been shown to be effective in reducing AF recurrence through significant reductions in systolic and diastolic blood pressure postablation,[49] providing further evidence as to the benefit of risk factor modification after catheter ablation.

MECHANISMS FOR EFFICACY OF RISK FACTOR MANAGEMENT BEFORE AND AFTER ABLATION

AF is a progressive disease in which the atrial cardiomyopathy gradually worsens with time. Clinically, this presents itself as a progression from paroxysmal AF to persistent and subsequently permanent forms of AF. The progressive nature of the atrial substrate underlying this natural progression of AF has been confirmed in atrial mapping studies; persistent AF is associated with larger left atrial dimensions, lower atrial regional voltages, increased proportion of low voltage areas, and increased proportion of complex signals (fractionated electrograms) within the left atrium.[50,51]

It is likely that these progressive changes explain the fact that catheter ablation of persistent AF is associated with higher attrition rates and poorer long-term maintenance of sinus rhythm in comparison to paroxysmal AF.[2] Cardiologists therefore favor a strategy of early ablation before the atrial substrate becomes unsalvageable and potentially unresponsive to ablation. RFM reverses the electrophysiologic remodeling of the left atrium and, therefore, improves the underlying atrial substrate prior to ablation, rendering the ablation procedure more likely to succeed (**Fig. 1**).

In addition, very late recurrences after ablation also relate to ongoing progression of the atrial substrate (**Fig. 1**). Despite AF ablation, the underlying atrial substrate has been shown to continue to evolve and progress, with further reductions in left atrial voltages and slowing of conduction seen at 10-month follow-up.[52] Recent data suggest that progression of atrial substrate may be linked to AF recurrence after ablation with new atrial fibrosis identified on late gadolinium enhancement magnetic resonance imaging (LGE-MRI) associated with increased risk of AF recurrence.[53] Furthermore, in a patient population with recurrent AF after pulmonary vein isolation, anatomic-based substrate ablation has been shown to improve long-term freedom from recurrence.[54] These studies highlight the importance of atrial substrate progression in AF recurrence after ablation and suggest that prevention or reversal of this progression both before and after ablation, therefore, is likely to improve long-term outcomes of AF ablation.

AGGRESSIVE RISK FACTOR MANAGEMENT REVERSES NATURAL PROGRESSION OF ATRIAL FIBRILLATION

Although antiarrhythmic medications and ablation have not been shown to reverse the natural

Table 4
Effect of RFM after ablation on long-term outcomes of AF ablation

Study	Type of Study	Postablation Intervention	Population	Changes in Risk Factors	Average Duration of Follow-up (months)	Number of Procedures	Outcomes
Pathak et al,[7] 2014 (ARREST-AF)	Cohort	Aggressive RFM	AF patients with BMI >27 kg/m_2 • 61 RFM • 88 standard care	RFM group • More weight reduction • Improved blood pressure control • Improved blood sugar control • Reduced sleep apnea	41.9	1.6 ± 0.7	• Reduced AF symptom burden ($P<.001$) • Improved arrhythmia-free survival—87% arrhythmia-free in RFM group vs 17% in control group (<0.001)
Pokushalov et al,[49] 2012	Randomized controlled trial	Renal artery denervation vs medical treatment	Symptomatic pAF/persAF refractory to 2 AADs with drug-resistant hypertension	Intervention group: BP improved from 181/97 to 156/87	12	1	Intervention group: 69% arrhythmia-free Control group: 29% arrhythmia-free ($P = .033$)

Details of studies investigating the impact of management (lifestyle, medical, and interventional) of individual and multiple risk factors after AF ablation procedure on AF ablation outcomes. AF, atrial fibrillation; AAD, antiarrhythmic drugs; BMI, body mass index; BP, blood pressure; RFM, risk factor management.

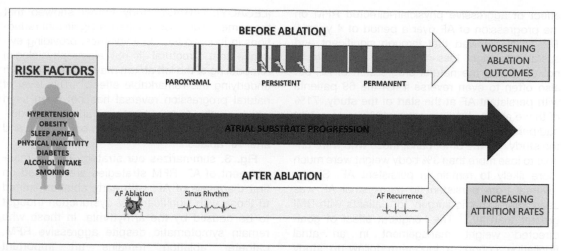

Fig. 1. Risk factors worsen AF ablation outcomes before and after ablation through their effect on atrial substrate. Before ablation, the presence of uncontrolled risk factors results in progression of the atrial substrate, progression from paroxysmal to persistent AF and therefore worsened long-term ablation outcomes. Risk factors continue to have the same effect on atrial substrate even after ablation, resulting in increased rates of attrition and AF recurrence.

progression of AF, RFM shows significant promise (**Fig. 2**). A recent study exploring the risk factors underlying AF progression showed that independent risk factors for progression included BMI, systolic blood pressure, and low physical activity.[55]

The PREVEntion and regReSsive Effect of weight-loss and risk factor modification on Atrial Fibrillation (REVERSE-AF) study investigated the

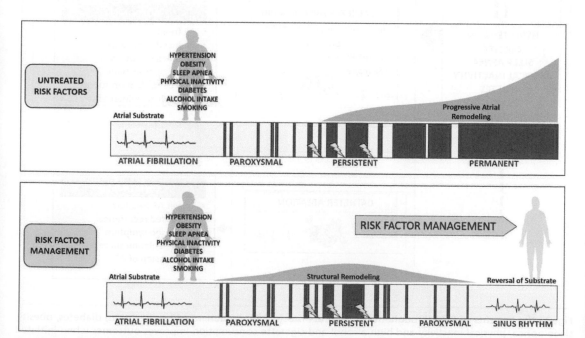

Fig. 2. The relationship between untreated risk factors, atrial remodeling, and clinical AF progression. Untreated risk factors are associated with structural and electrophysiologic remodeling of the atria, resulting in progression of AF and worsened clinical outcomes. RFM prevents and reverses atrial remodeling, reducing and reversing AF progression, thereby improving AF outcomes.

effect of aggressive physician-directed RFM on the progression of AF over a period of 4 years.[8] The study showed that through significant and sustained weight loss, individuals were able to not only slow the natural progression of AF but also often to even reverse it. Of the 69 patients with persistent AF at the start of the study, 71% of those able to lose more than 10% body weight had paroxysmal rather persistent AF by the end of the study. On the other hand, those who were unable to lose more than 3% body weight were much more likely to remain in persistent AF. Similar reversal from persistent to paroxysmal AF was seen after bariatric surgery for patients with BMI greater than 40.[41] The Longterm effect of goal-directed weight management in an atrial fibrillation cohort: a long-term follow-up study

(LEGACY). LEGACY study further showed that the same weight loss resulted in significant reductions in indexed left atrial volumes, providing evidence that structural (if not electrophysiologic) remodeling of the left atrium may be a mechanism underlying this remarkable effect.[10] This level of natural progression reversal has not been seen with any other form of treatment and likely underlies the improved outcomes seen both before and after AF ablation.

Fig. 3. summarizes our strategy for the management of AF. RFM strategies are initiated on first diagnosis of AF, with early ablation limited to those with significant LV dysfunction thought to be caused by the arrhythmia. In those who remain symptomatic despite aggressive RFM, catheter ablation remains an important

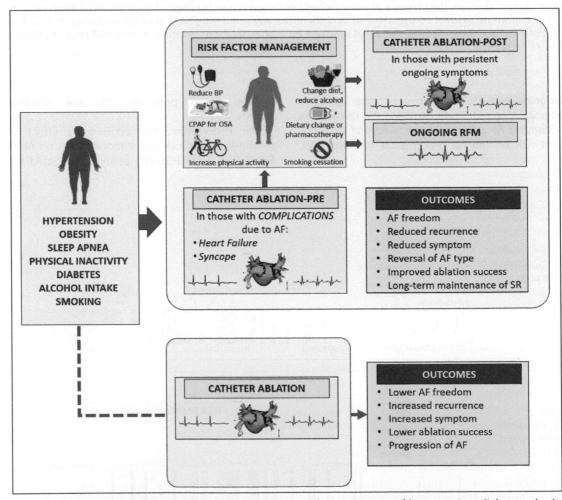

Fig. 3. The benefits of RFM throughout the natural history of AF. Treatment of hypertension, diabetes, obesity, sleep apnea, physical inactivity and high alcohol and cigarette consumption improves outcomes when initiated both before and after ablation. Ablation remains important in those with impaired LV function or syncope due to AF and in those who remain symptomatic despite aggressive RFM. However, the absence of adjunctive RFM for these patients results in worse catheter ablation outcomes. AF, atrial fibrillation; CPAP, continuous positive airway pressure; OSA, obstructive sleep apnea; RFM, risk factor management; SR, sinus rhythm.

component of the management strategy. However, RFM continues post-ablation to optimise the benefits of ablation. We have shown that this strategy is associated with improved long-term freedom from AF, reduced recurrences after ablation and reduced symptoms associated with AF.[7,10]

PRACTICALITIES OF RISK FACTOR MANAGEMENT—INTEGRATED CARE MODELS FOR ATRIAL FIBRILLATION

The clear cost-effectiveness of RFM programs for health care systems has been demonstrated in the Cost-Effectiveness and Clinical Effectiveness of the Risk Factor Management Clinic in Atrial Fibrillation (CENT) study.[9] This study showed that despite the increased costs associated with a more intense follow-up regime, the overall cost-effectiveness weighed heavily toward aggressive RFM, due to reductions in the need for additional medications or interventions and reduced hospital admissions and unplanned specialist clinic visits in the long-term. Despite this overwhelming evidence supporting RFM, however, the practicalities of aggressive RFM in traditional health care models are not straightforward.

In order to improve RFM in large patient populations, specialist multidisciplinary, fully integrated AF clinics have been shown to be effective. These clinics provide a standardized focus on RFM in addition to the traditional medical and interventional approach to AF. Whilst the cardiologist remains essential in directing and coordinating an overall management strategy, these clinics rely on the involvement of other medical and healthcare practitioners including specialist AF nurses, endocrinologists, sleep physicians, exercise physiologists and pharmacists. Involvement of these specialists allows for holistic assessment, monitoring, and treatment of all the risk factors known to contribute significantly to AF, which could not be reasonably carried out by a cardiologist alone. The positive effect of such clinics in attaining good RFM and AF outcomes has now been proved in several studies.[7–10,43]

Although the medical management of comorbid conditions is important, it is changes in patient behavior and lifestyle that are the cornerstone of RFM and essential for long-term success. A patient-centered approach to educate, encourage, and motivate patients toward a significant and long-lasting change in lifestyle, therefore, is critical. Changing habitual practice is a long process in which strong rapport with the patient must be built and personal motivations for change explored. Joint decision making to develop action plans with achievable targets is the next step toward sustained behavioral change. It is in these respects that the multidisciplinary AF team plays its most valuable role. The expert and interpersonal skills offered by the AF specialist nurse, in particular, are critical, and this has been confirmed through several studies, which have shown the importance of integrated care in AF.[56–58]

SUMMARY

Cardiovascular risk factors are critical in the development of the underlying abnormal atrial substrate and progression of AF. Whilst interventional AF ablation continues to improve in efficacy and safety, long-term attrition due to substrate progression is a significant drawback. There is increasing evidence to suggest that systematic and aggressive RFM can reduce this attrition through reversing the natural progression of AF and thereby improve ablation outcomes. Aggressive RFM is effective when initiated both before and after catheter ablation. Comprehensive RFM and integrated care clinics for AF are both successful and cost-effective. These multidisciplinary clinics allow improved patient education and better risk factor control through the delivery of tailored and bespoke management plans.

DISCLOSURE

Financial disclosures: Dr D. Lau is supported by the Robert J. Craig Lectureship from the University of Adelaide. Dr P. Sanders is supported by a Practitioner Fellowships from the National Health and Medical Research Council of Australia and by the National Heart Foundation of Australia.

Conflict of interest disclosures: Dr P. Sanders reports having served on the advisory board of Medtronic, Abbott Medical, Boston Scientific, CathRx, and PaceMate. Dr P. Sanders reports that the University of Adelaide has received on his behalf lecture and/or consulting fees from Medtronic, Abbott Medical, and Boston Scientific. Dr P. Sanders reports that the University of Adelaide has received on his behalf research funding from Medtronic, Abbott Medical, Boston Scientific, and MicroPort.

REFERENCES

1. Gallagher C, Hendriks JM, Giles L, et al. Increasing trends in hospitalisations due to atrial fibrillation in Australia from 1993 to 2013. Heart 2019;105(17): 1358–63.
2. Ganesan AN, Shipp NJ, Brooks AG, et al. Long-term outcomes of catheter ablation of atrial fibrillation: a

systematic review and meta-analysis. J Am Heart Assoc 2013;2(2):e004549.

3. Medi C, Sparks PB, Morton JB, et al. Pulmonary vein antral isolation for paroxysmal atrial fibrillation: results from long-term follow-up. J Cardiovasc Electrophysiol 2011;22(2):137–41.

4. Ouyang F, Tilz R, Chun J, et al. Long-term results of catheter ablation in paroxysmal atrial fibrillation: lessons from a 5-year follow-up. Circulation 2010; 122(23):2368–77.

5. Steinberg JS, Palekar R, Sichrovsky T, et al. Very long-term outcome after initially successful catheter ablation of atrial fibrillation. Heart Rhythm 2014; 11(5):771–6.

6. Weerasooriya R, Khairy P, Litalien J, et al. Catheter ablation for atrial fibrillation: are results maintained at 5 years of follow-up? J Am Coll Cardiol 2011; 57(2):160–6.

7. Pathak RK, Middeldorp ME, Lau DH, et al. Aggressive risk factor reduction study for atrial fibrillation and implications for the outcome of ablation: the ARREST-AF cohort study. J Am Coll Cardiol 2014; 64(21):2222–31.

8. Middeldorp ME, Pathak RK, Meredith M, et al. PREVEntion and regReSsive Effect of weight-loss and risk factor modification on Atrial Fibrillation: the REVERSE-AF study. Europace 2018;20(12): 1929–35.

9. Pathak RK, Evans M, Middeldorp ME, et al. Cost-effectiveness and clinical effectiveness of the risk factor management clinic in atrial fibrillation: the CENT study. JACC Clin Electrophysiol 2017;3(5): 436–47.

10. Pathak RK, Middeldorp ME, Meredith M, et al. Long-term effect of goal-directed weight management in an atrial fibrillation cohort: a long-term follow-up study (LEGACY). J Am Coll Cardiol 2015;65(20): 2159–69.

11. Benjamin EJ, Levy D, Vaziri SM, et al. Independent risk factors for atrial fibrillation in a population-based cohort. The Framingham Heart Study. JAMA 1994;271(11):840–4.

12. Okin PM, Hille DA, Larstorp AC, et al. Effect of lower on-treatment systolic blood pressure on the risk of atrial fibrillation in hypertensive patients. Hypertension 2015;66(2):368–73.

13. Lau DH, Mackenzie L, Kelly DJ, et al. Hypertension and atrial fibrillation: evidence of progressive atrial remodeling with electrostructural correlate in a conscious chronically instrumented ovine model. Heart Rhythm 2010;7(9):1282–90.

14. Lau DH, Mackenzie L, Kelly DJ, et al. Short-term hypertension is associated with the development of atrial fibrillation substrate: a study in an ovine hypertensive model. Heart Rhythm 2010;7(3): 396–404.

15. Lau DH, Shipp NJ, Kelly DJ, et al. Atrial arrhythmia in ageing spontaneously hypertensive rats: unraveling the substrate in hypertension and ageing. PLoS One 2013;8(8):e72416.

16. Aune D, Feng T, Schlesinger S, et al. Diabetes mellitus, blood glucose and the risk of atrial fibrillation: a systematic review and meta-analysis of cohort studies. J Diabetes Complications 2018;32(5): 501–11.

17. Kato T, Yamashita T, Sekiguchi A, et al. AGEs-RAGE system mediates atrial structural remodeling in the diabetic rat. J Cardiovasc Electrophysiol 2008; 19(4):415–20.

18. Liu C, Fu H, Li J, et al. Hyperglycemia aggravates atrial interstitial fibrosis, ionic remodeling and vulnerability to atrial fibrillation in diabetic rabbits. Anadolu Kardiyol Derg 2012;12(7):543–50.

19. Wong CX, Sullivan T, Sun MT, et al. Obesity and the risk of incident, post-operative, and post-ablation atrial fibrillation: a meta-analysis of 626,603 individuals in 51 studies. JACC Clin Electrophysiol 2015; 1(3):139–52.

20. Abed HS, Samuel CS, Lau DH, et al. Obesity results in progressive atrial structural and electrical remodeling: implications for atrial fibrillation. Heart Rhythm 2013;10(1):90–100.

21. Mahajan R, Lau DH, Brooks AG, et al. Electrophysiological, electroanatomical, and structural remodeling of the atria as consequences of sustained obesity. J Am Coll Cardiol 2015;66(1):1–11.

22. Munger TM, Dong YX, Masaki M, et al. Electrophysiological and hemodynamic characteristics associated with obesity in patients with atrial fibrillation. J Am Coll Cardiol 2012;60(9):851–60.

23. Wong CX, Abed HS, Molaee P, et al. Pericardial fat is associated with atrial fibrillation severity and ablation outcome. J Am Coll Cardiol 2011;57(17): 1745–51.

24. Hatem SN, Sanders P. Epicardial adipose tissue and atrial fibrillation. Cardiovasc Res 2014;102(2): 205–13.

25. Youssef I, Kamran H, Yacoub M, et al. Obstructive sleep apnea as a risk factor for atrial fibrillation: a meta-analysis. J Sleep Disord Ther 2018;7(1) [pii:282].

26. Linz D, Schotten U, Neuberger HR, et al. Negative tracheal pressure during obstructive respiratory events promotes atrial fibrillation by vagal activation. Heart Rhythm 2011;8(9):1436–43.

27. Holtstrand Hjalm H, Fu M, Hansson PO, et al. Association between left atrial enlargement and obstructive sleep apnea in a general population of 71-year-old men. J Sleep Res 2018;27(2):252–8.

28. Iwasaki YK, Kato T, Xiong F, et al. Atrial fibrillation promotion with long-term repetitive obstructive sleep apnea in a rat model. J Am Coll Cardiol 2014;64(19): 2013–23.

29. Gallagher C, Hendriks JML, Elliott AD, et al. Alcohol and incident atrial fibrillation - a systematic review and meta-analysis. Int J Cardiol 2017;246:46–52.

30. Voskoboinik A, Wong G, Lee G, et al. Moderate alcohol consumption is associated with atrial electrical and structural changes: insights from high-density left atrial electroanatomic mapping. Heart Rhythm 2019;16(2):251–9.

31. Mandyam MC, Vedantham V, Scheinman MM, et al. Alcohol and vagal tone as triggers for paroxysmal atrial fibrillation. Am J Cardiol 2012;110(3):364–8.

32. Tolstrup JS, Wium-Andersen MK, Orsted DD, et al. Alcohol consumption and risk of atrial fibrillation: observational and genetic estimates of association. Eur J Prev Cardiol 2016;23(14):1514–23.

33. McManus DD, Yin X, Gladstone R, et al. Alcohol consumption, left atrial diameter, and atrial fibrillation. J Am Heart Assoc 2016;5(9) [pii:e004060].

34. Chamberlain AM, Agarwal SK, Folsom AR, et al. Smoking and incidence of atrial fibrillation: results from the Atherosclerosis Risk in Communities (ARIC) study. Heart Rhythm 2011;8(8):1160–6.

35. Frost L, Hune LJ, Vestergaard P. Overweight and obesity as risk factors for atrial fibrillation or flutter: the Danish Diet, Cancer, and Health Study. Am J Med 2005;118(5):489–95.

36. Smith JG, Platonov PG, Hedblad B, et al. Atrial fibrillation in the Malmo Diet and Cancer study: a study of occurrence, risk factors and diagnostic validity. Eur J Epidemiol 2010;25(2):95–102.

37. Albertsen IE, Rasmussen LH, Lane DA, et al. The impact of smoking on thromboembolism and mortality in patients with incident atrial fibrillation: insights from the Danish Diet, Cancer, and Health study. Chest 2014;145(3):559–66.

38. Mohanty S, Mohanty P, Tamaki M, et al. Differential association of exercise intensity with risk of atrial fibrillation in men and women: evidence from a meta-analysis. J Cardiovasc Electrophysiol 2016; 27(9):1021–9.

39. Mozaffarian D, Furberg CD, Psaty BM, et al. Physical activity and incidence of atrial fibrillation in older adults: the cardiovascular health study. Circulation 2008;118(8):800–7.

40. Jin MN, Yang PS, Song C, et al. Physical activity and risk of atrial fibrillation: a nationwide cohort study in general population. Sci Rep 2019;9(1):13270.

41. Donnellan E, Wazni OM, Elshazly M, et al. Impact of Bariatric Surgery on Atrial Fibrillation Type. Circ Arrhythm Electrophysiol 2020;13(2):e007626.

42. Fein AS, Shvilkin A, Shah D, et al. Treatment of obstructive sleep apnea reduces the risk of atrial fibrillation recurrence after catheter ablation. J Am Coll Cardiol 2013;62(4):300–5.

43. Pathak RK, Elliott A, Middeldorp ME, et al. Impact of cardiorespiratory fitness on arrhythmia recurrence in obese individuals with atrial fibrillation:

the CARDIO-FIT study. J Am Coll Cardiol 2015; 66(9):985–96.

44. Donnellan E, Wazni OM, Kanj M, et al. Association between pre-ablation bariatric surgery and atrial fibrillation recurrence in morbidly obese patients undergoing atrial fibrillation ablation. Europace 2019; 21(10):1476–83.

45. Patel D, Mohanty P, Di Biase L, et al. Safety and efficacy of pulmonary vein antral isolation in patients with obstructive sleep apnea: the impact of continuous positive airway pressure. Circ Arrhythm Electrophysiol 2010;3(5):445–51.

46. Santoro F, Di Biase L, Trivedi C, et al. Impact of uncontrolled hypertension on atrial fibrillation ablation outcome. JACC Clin Electrophysiol 2015;1(3): 164–73.

47. Parkash R, Wells GA, Sapp JL, et al. Effect of aggressive blood pressure control on the recurrence of atrial fibrillation after catheter ablation: a randomized, open-label clinical trial (SMAC-AF [Substrate Modification with Aggressive Blood Pressure Control]). Circulation 2017;135(19):1788–98.

48. Balk EM, Garlitski AC, Alsheikh-Ali AA, et al. Predictors of atrial fibrillation recurrence after radiofrequency catheter ablation: a systematic review. J Cardiovasc Electrophysiol 2010;21(11): 1208–16.

49. Pokushalov E, Romanov A, Corbucci G, et al. A randomized comparison of pulmonary vein isolation with versus without concomitant renal artery denervation in patients with refractory symptomatic atrial fibrillation and resistant hypertension. J Am Coll Cardiol 2012;60(13):1163–70.

50. Teh AW, Kalman JM, Kistler PM, et al. Prevalence of fractionated electrograms in the coronary sinus: comparison between patients with persistent or paroxysmal atrial fibrillation and a control population. Heart Rhythm 2010;7(9):1200–4.

51. Teh AW, Kistler PM, Lee G, et al. Electroanatomic remodeling of the left atrium in paroxysmal and persistent atrial fibrillation patients without structural heart disease. J Cardiovasc Electrophysiol 2012;23(3): 232–8.

52. Teh AW, Kistler PM, Lee G, et al. Long-term effects of catheter ablation for lone atrial fibrillation: progressive atrial electroanatomic substrate remodeling despite successful ablation. Heart Rhythm 2012; 9(4):473–80.

53. Kheirkhahan M, Baher A, Goldooz M, et al. Left atrial fibrosis progression detected by LGE-MRI after ablation of atrial fibrillation. Pacing Clin Electrophysiol 2019.

54. Shah S, Barakat AF, Saliba WI, et al. Recurrent atrial fibrillation after initial long-term ablation success: electrophysiological findings and outcomes of repeat ablation procedures. Circ Arrhythm Electrophysiol 2018;11(4):e005785.

55. Blum S, Aeschbacher S, Meyre P, et al. Incidence and predictors of atrial fibrillation progression. J Am Heart Assoc 2019;8(20):e012554.

56. Carter L, Gardner M, Magee K, et al. An integrated management approach to atrial fibrillation. J Am Heart Assoc 2016;5(1) [pii:e002950].

57. Hendriks JM, de Wit R, Crijns HJ, et al. Nurse-led care vs. usual care for patients with atrial fibrillation: results of a randomized trial of integrated chronic care vs. routine clinical care in ambulatory patients with atrial fibrillation. Eur Heart J 2012;33(21): 2692–9.

58. Stewart S, Ball J, Horowitz JD, et al. Standard versus atrial fibrillation-specific management strategy (SAFETY) to reduce recurrent admission and prolong survival: pragmatic, multicentre, randomised controlled trial. Lancet 2015;385(9970):775–84.

59. Huxley RR, Lopez FL, Folsom AR, et al. Absolute and attributable risks of atrial fibrillation in relation to optimal and borderline risk factors: the Atherosclerosis Risk in Communities (ARIC) study. Circulation 2011;123(14):1501–8.

60. Asad Z, Abbas M, Javed I, et al. Obesity is associated with incident atrial fibrillation independent of gender: a meta-analysis. J Cardiovasc Electrophysiol 2018;29(5):725–32.

61. Aune D, Schlesinger S, Norat T, et al. Tobacco smoking and the risk of atrial fibrillation: a systematic review and meta-analysis of prospective studies. Eur J Prev Cardiol 2018;25(13):1437–51.

62. Mohanty S, Mohanty P, Natale V, et al. Impact of weight loss on ablation outcome in obese patients with longstanding persistent atrial fibrillation. J Cardiovasc Electrophysiol 2018;29(2): 246–53.

63. Bazan V, Grau N, Valles E, et al. Obstructive sleep apnea in patients with typical atrial flutter: prevalence and impact on arrhythmia control outcome. Chest 2013;143(5):1277–83.

64. Jongnarangsin K, Chugh A, Good E, et al. Body mass index, obstructive sleep apnea, and outcomes of catheter ablation of atrial fibrillation. J Cardiovasc Electrophysiol 2008;19(7):668–72.

How, When, and Why
High-Density Mapping of Atrial Fibrillation

Santhisri Kodali, MD[a], Pasquale Santangeli, MD, PhD[b],*

KEYWORDS

- High-density mapping • Atrial fibrillation • Catheter ablation

KEY POINTS

- Compared with traditional PBP mapping, HD mapping presents opportunities to enhance delineation of atrial fibrillation (AF) substrate, greatly improve the efficiency of the mapping procedure without sacrificing safety, and afford new mechanistic insights regarding AF.
- Innovations in hardware, software algorithms, and development of novel multielectrode catheters have enabled HD mapping to be feasible and reliable.
- Further refinements anticipated in the future in automated HD mapping include evolution of noncontact methodologies and artificial intelligence to supplant current techniques.

INTRODUCTION

Since its inception, percutaneous catheter ablation including pulmonary vein (PV) isolation has progressed to become a cornerstone of treatment of symptomatic atrial fibrillation (AF). This advance in treatment was made following the seminal study that demonstrated ectopic foci originating from the PVs represented greater than 90% of AF triggers.[1] Non-PV triggers of AF, such as the posterior wall, superior vena cava, left atrial appendage, coronary sinus (CS), ligament of Marshall, and right atrial triggers, have also been demonstrated to promote genesis of AF.[2–4] Although PV isolation has been an acceptable strategy to address paroxysmal AF, the outcomes for persistent AF have been significantly less favorable and often, additional substrate modification is performed.[5,6] It is therefore clear that improving spatiotemporal resolution of voltage mapping is pivotal to better address the underlying substrate. For the interventional electrophysiologist, ablative success is highly dependent on the rendering of an accurate geometric and electrical representation of the heart by the three-dimensional (3D) electroanatomic mapping (EAM) system and mapping catheter. In particular, the advent of novel multielectrode catheters coupled with advances in nonfluoroscopic navigational EAM systems has enabled the performance of high-density (HD) mapping and consequently, the tackling of increasingly complex and challenging arrhythmias.

There are certain situations in which HD mapping is especially useful and even indispensable to optimize the success of ablation. In this review, we describe the approach to HD mapping of AF and importantly, why it should be a fundamental element of the interventional electrophysiologist's toolbox.

GENERAL APPROACH TO MAPPING OF ATRIAL FIBRILLATION

Before the ablation procedure, patients are typically maintained on either uninterrupted or

[a] Cardiac Electrophysiology, The University of Texas Medical Branch, 301 8th Street, Galveston, TX 77550, USA;
[b] Cardiac Electrophysiology, Hospital of the University of Pennsylvania, 3400 Spruce Street, 9 Founders Pavilion, Philadelphia, PA 19104, USA
* Corresponding author.
E-mail address: pasquale.santangeli@pennmedicine.upenn.edu

Card Electrophysiol Clin 12 (2020) 155–165
https://doi.org/10.1016/j.ccep.2020.02.004
1877-9182/20/© 2020 Elsevier Inc. All rights reserved.

minimally interrupted oral anticoagulation. Antiarrhythmics are discontinued at least five half-lives before the procedure, with the exception of amiodarone. The procedure is performed under general anesthesia and an unfractionated heparin infusion is maintained to keep the goal serum activated clotting time greater than 300 seconds. A decapolar catheter is placed in the CS to provide stable reference signals for mapping. Intracardiac echocardiography is used to guide transseptal punctures and catheter positioning, permit direct visualization of structures, and monitor for potential complications. Following transseptal puncture, we find the use of high-frequency, low-volume ventilation when available to be helpful in improving catheter contact and stability. A 3D electroanatomic map is then constructed of the left atrium (LA) and displayed via a nonfluoroscopic navigational mapping system (eg, CARTO [Biosense Webster, Diamond Bar, CA], Precision [Abbott, St. Paul, MN], Rhythmia HDx [Boston Scientific, Cambridge, MA]). Initially, the approach to LA mapping was accomplished via a roving ablation catheter with a 3.5-mm distal electrode tip and a sequential point-by-point (PBP) acquisition strategy.[7] Contemporary procedures, however, tend to use HD mapping systems and multielectrode mapping catheters. This is a natural consequence of the increased number of ablation procedures being carried out particularly in patients with persistent AF and complex structural heart disease whose underlying substrate demands more powerful mapping strategies and automated algorithms.

The fiber orientation pattern of the LA in addition to the remodeling that occurs over time because of AF contributes to development of the putative substrate and low-voltage regions. A recent study used cardiac MRI to corroborate prior observations of LA fiber orientation, demonstrating the predominant pattern of LA fibers transitioning from longitudinal at the roof to circular at the PVs. The LA fibers of the endocardial versus epicardial layers were also found to be perpendicular to each other except at the lateral wall and roof, where the angles remained constant.[8] Considerable asynchrony between the endocardial and epicardial surfaces may occur during AF, providing a route for transmural fibrillatory conduction.[9]

Assessment of atrial fibrosis by late gadolinium enhancement cardiac MRI is constrained by its spatial resolution, the relative thinness of the LA wall, and lack of standardized acquisition sequences. Furthermore, AF substrate that is electrically passive under baseline conditions and not perceived during initial voltage mapping may be unmasked when subjected to electrophysiologic stress because of anisotropy, functional block and reentry, decreased conduction velocity, and dispersion of refractoriness. When mapping the LA, higher fidelity signal acquisition revealing electrogram characteristics, such as fractionation, low amplitude, and moment of local depolarization, become important in defining the substrate and augmenting knowledge of the mechanisms facilitating AF generation and perpetuation.

TECHNICAL CONSIDERATIONS OF VOLTAGE MAPPING

Voltage mapping allows characterization of electrical wavefront propagation by measurement of local activation times (LAT) with respect to a reference signal and also permits delineation of AF substrate by relying on voltage amplitude as an electrical surrogate for tissue health. Both bipolar and unipolar voltage signals are practically useful in this regard and serve a fundamental role in treating AF and other atrial arrhythmias (ie, atrial flutter, atrial tachycardia) related to de novo fibrosis or proarrhythmia because of the effects of iatrogenic scar following prior AF ablation.

Unipolar signals assess differences in extracellular potential between the exploring electrode and a distant reference electrode. They are not directionally dependent and the steepest negative dV/dt has been found to be the best correlate of local tissue activation.[10,11] Unipolar electrograms are influenced by low-frequency signals, such as those of far-field origin and artifact and thus, may conceal low-amplitude electrograms.[12] Consequently, bipolar electrograms are frequently relied on and derived from extracellular potential differences between two closely spaced electrodes (ie, bipole). The closer the electrodes constituting a bipole are spaced, the more they approach the first derivative of the corresponding unipolar signal.[13] The bipolar electrogram is generated using differential amplifiers or postprocessing of unipolar signals corresponding to the bipole electrodes to cancel out most of the far-field components. The temporal offset of local depolarization between the electrodes then determines bipolar signal morphology. Bipolar signals are known to be subject to the following: (1) direction of wavefront propagation relative to the scanning pair of electrodes; (2) conduction velocity of the signal; (3) bipole orientation relative to the tissue surface (ie, angle of incidence); and (4) characteristics of the electrode pair itself including electrode size, interelectrode spacing,[14] and impedance. A study by Williams and colleagues[15] showed that the direction of wavefront activation in the LA (high right atrium and CS pacing) influenced the recorded bipolar voltage amplitude. More recent studies have revealed marked changes in fractionation, amplitude, and polarity of atrial bipolar electrograms and conduction velocities affecting the mapped atrial substrate patterns, resulting from CS versus left superior PV pacing and use of varying pacing drivetrains and coupled extrastimuli.[16,17] These investigations reinforce the directional weakness of bipolar signals. Directional dependence had been previously demonstrated in the ventricles as well.[18] The maximum amplitude or peak negative dV/dt of the bipolar signal may be used for LAT annotation.[19] However, low-amplitude, fractionated signals present a challenge because they require greater manual annotation and careful distinction must be made between near-field and far-field components. Moreover, use of a single fiducial point to determine LAT may not be sufficiently reliable and lead to creation of misleading maps. In addition, near-field signals from small islands or channels of viable myocytes may be obscured depending on the electrode characteristics and potential for far-field interference and interference caused by the inherent background noise of conventional mapping systems.

During AF ablation procedures, bipolar voltage mapping was traditionally performed using a sequential PBP strategy with a standard ablation catheter. This can provide information regarding contact force and decrease the probability of an area of "low voltage or scar" caused by inadequate tissue contact. However, it is a time-consuming process, limited in spatial resolution, and not well suited to nonsustained rhythms or those not hemodynamically tolerated. In addition, the larger electrode reduces sensitivity to low-amplitude signals falsely amplifying the size of low-voltage regions. The findings of Anter and colleagues[20] are in line with this, whereby a comparison between the 1-mm electrodes of the PentaRay mapping catheter with the 3.5-mm ThermoCool ablation catheter, Irvine, California was performed. Following sequential mapping, they found that in nondiseased atria, there was no significant difference in the amplitude of bipolar electrograms regardless of the catheter used. However, with respect to low-voltage (<0.5 mV) regions within diseased atria, the total bipolar low-voltage area was less, the mean bipolar amplitude greater, and discrete electrogram components sharper (increasing reliability of LAT annotation) with the PentaRay catheter. Moreover, pacing could be performed at a lower output with the multielectrode catheter because of increased current density at the tissue-electrode interface.[20] Similar findings regarding bipolar electrograms have been noted in an ovine ventricular infarct model focused on the effects of interelectrode spacing and a computational study examining the effect of wavefront angle and interelectrode spacing in a biodomain model of the human atrium.[21,22] Another observation has been the notable and intuitive reduction in mean bipolar electrogram amplitude during AF relative to sinus rhythm, demonstrated in prior studies.[23,24] However, the voltage amplitudes obtained may be further affected by a multitude of factors, such as atrial cycle length, a regular versus an everchanging wavefront direction, pacing site chosen, and the anatomic subregion within the atrium.[7,23,25] At present, no clear guideline exists regarding the best rhythm during which to perform mapping. Our own preference is to perform mapping in sinus rhythm whenever possible or pace the atrium slightly faster than the sinus rate. The operator should also keep in mind that low-voltage electrogram criteria during the procedure may need to be tailored based on the catheter bipole configuration.[26,27]

Although prior generations of EAM systems were technically capable of performing HD mapping with multielectrode catheters, it was a lengthy task fraught with the need for manual annotation following electrogram data collection, and was prone to error either by the operator or the system regarding appropriate acceptance or rejection of mapping data. The most recent HD mapping systems have made significant strides toward mitigating these issues through novel mapping methodology, hardware innovations, and automated software algorithms. In particular, uniquely shaped multielectrode catheters have been developed that can simultaneously acquire a significantly greater amount of data from a larger area with higher fidelity, reduce data interpolation, and undergo automated and rapid signal processing. The electrodes used are of low impedance to maximize the signal-to-noise ratio. However, given that contact force sensing is presently not available with dedicated multipolar mapping catheters, the operator must rely on surrogate markers, such as variance in electrode impedance to judge proximity to tissue. The following sections describe the major HD EAM systems along with their respective novel multielectrode mapping catheters.

HIGH-DENSITY MAPPING SYSTEMS
Rhythmia HDx

The Rhythmia HDx ultra-HD mapping system is used in conjunction with the bidirectional deflectable 64-electrode mini-basket Orion catheter (Boston Scientific). This novel catheter consists of eight splines and each spline carries eight electrodes of low impedance, a 0.4-mm^2 individual electrode surface area, and 2.5-mm electrode spacing measured center-to-center. The Rhythmia HDx system uses a combination of magnetic sensing (distal catheter tip) and impedance sensing (64 electrode basket array). It permits the automatic and rapid collection of multiple electrograms without a ceiling to the number of data points that can be acquired, without dependency on manual annotation, and with limited or no post-processing of electrogram data required afterward. Demarcation of bipolar low-voltage regions can be set less than 0.03 mV because the bipolar noise of the system is less than 0.01 mV. This noise floor, in addition to the basket catheter microelectrodes, has allowed for a new level of distinguishing heterogeneity within low-voltage regions. Selection of the appropriate potential for LAT annotation of multicomponent bipolar signals involves analysis of the relative timing of signals from neighboring tissue (at least two references) and the maximal negative dV/dt of the corresponding unipolar electrogram for comparison. The Lumipoint software module was introduced more recently and highlights regions of interesting signals on the electroanatomic map, such as fractionated, late, or double potentials, making it easier for the operator to home in on these areas. **Fig. 1** displays an example of a high-resolution activation map of the LA created with the Rhythmia HDx mapping system.

EnSite Precision

Multipolar HD mapping with the EnSite Precision system is accomplished with a variety of catheter configurations including linear, multispline, and circular catheters. The recently released Advisor HD Grid (Abbott) mapping catheter contains a grid shaped 4 × 4 equidistant array of electrodes distributed among four splines, with 3-mm interelectrode spacing, and a 1-mm^2 individual electrode surface area. The HD Grid was designed with the concept of omnipolar mapping, introduced by Deno and colleagues[28] as a method to more consistently assess the physiologic characteristics of the tissue being sampled. If the electrical wave is perpendicular to the measuring bipole, minimal voltage is detected, whereas it records a maximal amplitude if the bipole is parallel to the path of depolarization. To determine the direction of the traveling wave then, either the catheter would have to be rotated a full 360° or a priori knowledge of the activation pattern would be necessary to align the catheter with the propagating wave, both of which are impractical strategies. The idea of an omnipole involves interrogation of the local electrical field associated with an activation wavefront in all directions (ie, spatial derivative) surrounding a clique of closely spaced electrodes. In the same manner, orthogonal bipoles contained within adjacent cliques of electrodes are also interrogated to produce omnipolar electrograms in the region being sampled. This allows for a directionally agnostic measurement of voltage and activation direction from a single beat, unlike with traditional unipoles and bipoles. Studies involving animal models and humans have validated this concept and shown that even during AF, the measured maximal voltages are indeed much less susceptible to directionality, wavefront collision, and fractionation in the case of omnipolar electrograms relative to bipolar.[29–31] Nevertheless, the full utility of omnipolar electrograms remains to be explored in studies, including assessment of intramural scar. The EnSite Precision mapping system performs omnipolar mapping via The Best Duplicate algorithm.

The HD Grid catheter contains magnetic sensing technology, enabling the collection of impedance and magnetic points to create a more accurate geometry of the cardiac chamber being mapped and produce higher fidelity signals. In addition, the design and pliability of the HD Grid minimizes map distortion that was seen with prior circular mapping catheters and creates minimal ectopy. The EnSite Precision mapping system AutoMap module introduces the TurboMap feature for automatic annotation of signals (based on user prespecified criteria) and rapid data processing, nearly eliminating the need for post-processing of acquired data afterward. The Sparkle Map feature allows visualization of electrical propagation superimposed on the voltage map. **Fig. 2** illustrates an HD electroanatomic map of the right atrium and LA constructed with the EnSite Precision mapping system in the setting of atypical flutter.

CARTO 3

Multipolar mapping with the CARTO 3 platform is amenable to multiple catheter configurations, including a linear decapolar catheter, a circular catheter, and a multispline catheter (ie, PentaRay). The lattermost is the most commonly used catheter to execute atrial and ventricular HD mapping. The PentaRay bipole configuration is a radial array comprised of five splines with each spline carrying four 1-mm electrodes with 2-6-2 mm

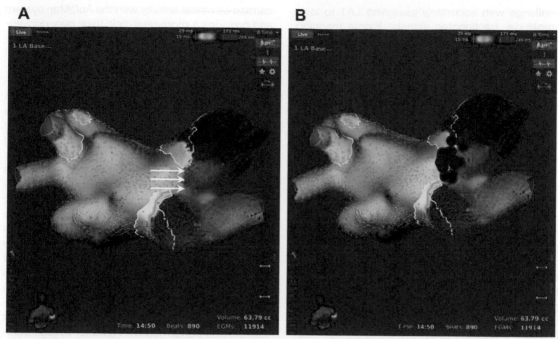

Fig. 1. Creation of a left atrial activation map with the Rhythmia HDx mapping system in a patient with persistent atrial fibrillation who had undergone prior pulmonary vein isolation. (*A*) The *white arrows* point to the conduction gap along the posterior right pulmonary vein carina as visualized by activation mapping. (*B*) Radiofrequency ablation lesions were applied as shown, resulting in reisolation of the right pulmonary veins.

interelectrode spacing and a deflectable tip (unidirectional up to 180°). The system relies on a hybrid of current and magnetic-based measurements to track catheter position. For timing annotation, the Biosense Webster Confidense module has been introduced to streamline the process of mapping by acquiring data only after meeting operator-prespecified criteria, and filtering of points based on tissue proximity. Reliable automated annotation became a feature and also incorporated unipolar and bipolar electrogram characteristics to validate mapping data. In addition, given the

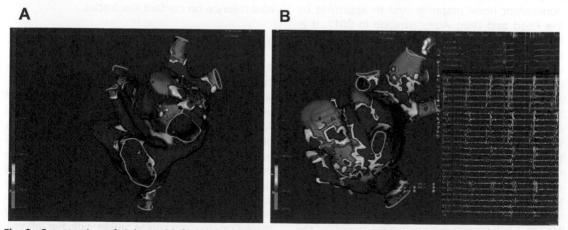

Fig. 2. Construction of right and left atrial voltage maps with the EnSite Precision mapping system in a patient with atypical atrial flutter and no prior history of catheter ablation or cardiac surgery. (*A*) Baseline bipolar voltage mapping during atrial flutter reveals significant fibrosis of the left atrium with relative sparing of the right atrium. (*B*) The HD Grid catheter, located within the left atrial appendage, reveals significantly delayed bipolar electrogram signals at baseline. Radiofrequency applications were ultimately placed from the left superior pulmonary vein to the left atrial appendage base with successful termination of the atrial flutter.

challenge with accurately assigning LAT to low-amplitude, fractionated signals, Ripple mapping was developed as an approach to dynamically track local myocardial voltage over time without sacrificing information from the bipolar electrogram and avoiding interpolation of unmapped regions.[32] More recently, the Coherent mapping module was introduced to the platform and attempts to resolve complex electrograms by taking into account all possible potentials comprising each electrogram, the derived conduction velocities based on LAT, and probability of nonconductivity based on physiologic assumptions to produce a color-coded vector map. The vector map displays the global activation pattern that represents the most stable and "coherent" mathematical solution to provide further insight into the arrhythmia mechanism.[33] **Fig. 3** displays HD voltage and Ripple maps of the LA created with the CARTO 3 mapping system to localize the region of conduction breakthrough. Finally, it should be mentioned that the OctaRay mapping catheter is a newer addition to the CARTO 3 platform and contains eight splines with six electrodes of surface area 0.9 mm^2 each and 2.5-mm interelectrode spacing. The catheter is still not available for clinical use, but it seems to be capable of creating even higher resolution maps than the PentaRay catheter and potentially better tissue apposition based on a porcine model.[34]

NONCONTACT HIGH-DENSITY MAPPING
Acutus

The AcQMap High Resolution Imaging and Mapping System (Acutus Medical, Carlsbad, CA) is a noncontact novel mapping system approved by the Food and Drug Administration in 2017. It is based on the concept of source modeling, first described in a seminal work in 2002.[35] In this context, macroscopic dipole density (DD) is considered a truer approximation of the source of cardiac electrical activity compared with traditionally measured voltage (although microscopic DD would be even more accurate, it remains unfeasible to measure with the currently available technology). Poisson equation represents the mathematical solution of the forward problem, determination of voltage corresponding to a known macroscopic DD. However, because cardiac electrical activity would ideally be modeled by the best source approximation possible, the mathematical inverse problem of deriving macroscopic DD from a measured voltage arises. It is the solution to this problem, via application of an inverse algorithm to Poisson equation, that is the fundamental basis for real-time modeling of

cardiac electrical activity with the AcQMap system and provides a more near-field view over conventional voltage mapping.[36] The AcQMap 3D Imaging and Mapping Catheter (Acutus Medical) contains six splines arranged in a spheroid configuration, with each spline containing eight mini ultrasound transducers and interspersed with eight low-impedance electrodes. The system is able to recreate a high-quality ultrasound reconstruction of the atrium within minutes. Noncontact sensing within the cardiac chamber, with a sampling rate of up to 150,000 biopotentials per second, is used to obtain voltage information and derive macroscopic DD for spatial and temporal display on the rendered 3D electroanatomic map. With the most recent version, contact mapping does remain an option if the operator prefers. The UNCOVER-AF prospective nonrandomized trial was recently performed to assess the effectiveness of the AcQMap system in patients with persistent AF undergoing first time catheter ablation. Thus far, the results seem to be consistent with studies performed with contact voltage mapping methodologies.[37] Nevertheless, randomized controlled trials are required to better assess the impact on clinical outcomes. **Fig. 4** illustrates an electroanatomic map of the LA constructed using the AcQMap system; the color-coded yellow and green regions represent sites of either localized irregular or rotational activity that may be targeted for ablation. Although further technological development is merited, the AcQMap system represents an important step forward because noncontact mapping systems offer the possibility of instantaneously determining global activation patterns of the entire cardiac chamber and obviates reliance on contact electrodes.

BENEFITS OF HIGH-DENSITY MAPPING

Although patients with persistent and long-standing persistent AF present an especially challenging substrate and stand to benefit the most from HD mapping, even patients with paroxysmal AF have been shown to harbor preexisting fibrosis of the LA and thus would also benefit from this technology. A greater scar burden has been commensurate with worse outcomes following catheter ablation of AF,[38–40] underscoring the importance of accurate electrogram data registration and creation of maps with high spatiotemporal resolution to accurately guide ablative efforts. Before the era of HD mapping, there was a significantly greater likelihood of regions on the LA voltage map erroneously appearing electrically silent or harboring low voltage, thus confounding the delineation of the AF substrate, identification of

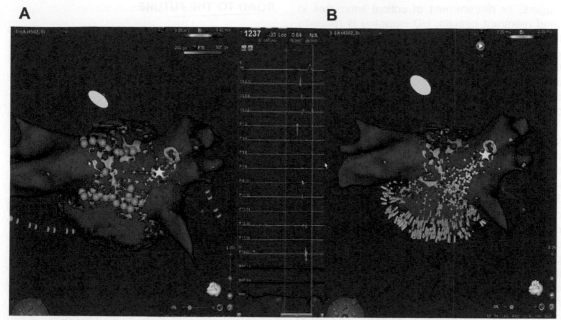

Fig. 3. Construction of left atrial voltage and Ripple maps with the CARTO 3 mapping system in a patient with persistent atrial fibrillation who had undergone prior pulmonary vein isolation. (*A*) Following posterior wall isolation, signals in the right superior pulmonary vein recorded by the PentaRay catheter revealed the site of reconnection as shown. The *yellow star* marks the site of right superior pulmonary vein isolation in both panels. (*B*) Ripple mapping illustrates slowed conduction into the right superior pulmonary vein, consistent with the eventual site of successful ablation.

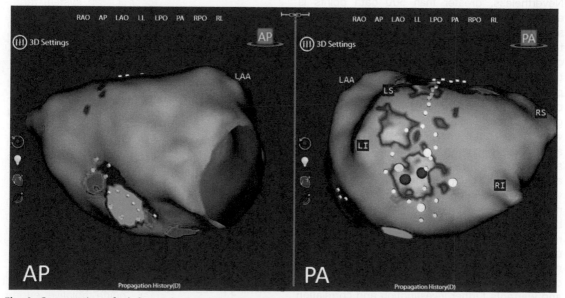

Fig. 4. Construction of a left atrial anatomic map with the ACUTUS system. The system is able to recreate a high-quality ultrasound reconstruction of the atrium within minutes using a dedicated catheter. In addition, analysis of repetitive AF activation patterns using dipole density mapping is possible with noncontact sensing within the cardiac chamber (sites highlighted in *yellow* and *green*). These sites may represent additional nonpulmonary vein targets for ablation. AP, anterior-posterior projection; LAA, left atrial appendage; PA, posterior-anterior projection.

triggers, or discernment of critical isthmuses in atrial reentrant circuits. HD mapping is requisite to visualize heterogeneity within regions of low-voltage, residual PV reconnection, gaps within the ablation lesion set, otherwise concealed low-amplitude PV signal propagation, and areas of complex potentials and slowed or rotatory conduction potentially critical for AF maintenance.[41,42]

HD mapping has been demonstrated to be as safe as conventional PBP mapping in the setting of AF[43] and has maintained safety and efficacy among a diverse spectrum of cardiac arrhythmias as demonstrated in the multicenter prospective TRUE HD study.[44] Patients with congenital heart disease are especially prone to arrhythmias caused by preexisting substrate, altered anatomy, and as a sequela of surgical or interventional procedures.[45] The effectiveness of HD mapping in patients with moderate to severe complex congenital heart disease has been illustrated by Alken and colleagues.[46] Not surprisingly, poorer clinical outcomes following catheter ablation of atrial tachycardia were associated with a greater preexistent low-voltage region in another investigation.[47]

LIMITATIONS OF HIGH-DENSITY MAPPING

There is no clear consensus on the density of points on the electroanatomic map that are needed to meet the definition of HD mapping. Nevertheless, greater than 500 data points is acceptable and suffice to say, the greater the density of points collected, the better the spatial and temporal resolution will be. However, a pitfall of collecting an overabundance of points is related to the potential for incorrect annotation and interpolation in the surrounding regions. Thus, it still behooves the operator to manually check electrogram data particularly if the map does not fit with what is physiologically known or the expected arrhythmia mechanism. In addition, if reentrant atrial circuits are visually seen, activation mapping alone may not clearly distinguish passively activated regions; entrainment mapping is a fundamental adjunct in this regard and should always be considered.[48] Current mapping techniques rely on static voltage mapping, which may fail to unmask dormant substrate or drivers of AF. Dynamic voltage attenuation is a strategy to partially overcome the limitations of bipolar electrograms and warrants further investigation and correlation with cardiac MRI.[17] Moreover, a limitation of contact HD mapping is the required sequential collection of electrogram data, making it less suited for assessing instantaneous global activation patterns relative to a noncontact mapping approach.

ROAD TO THE FUTURE

In recent years, appreciation of the complex 3D atrial architecture has grown. Although current clinically available HD mapping technologies focus on studying the atrial endocardial surface and also support epicardial surface mapping, this only reveals part of the picture. In particular, the intramural layer represents a dimension that thus far remains hazy and serves as an important link to mechanistic insights of AF generation, sustenance, and abolition. The current yield of noncontact methodologies applying the mathematical inverse solution to sophisticated algorithms (based on prespecified physiologic constraints) to perform noninvasive HD mapping has largely been confined to the experimental realm. This is complicated by the fact that the amplitude of atrial signals is much lower relative to ventricular, rendering inverse reconstruction more challenging to implement. In the near future, it is hoped that noninvasive mapping will enter clinical prime time and enable real-time visualization of 3D substrate and global activation patterns.

A modality that has the capability to provide significantly higher spatial and temporal resolution over that of multielectrode array mapping is optical mapping. It resolves action potentials and transient calcium currents via a combination of voltage-sensitive dyes and an optical sensor or high-speed cameras.[49] Additionally, it would also enable visualization of wavefront propagation patterns even during applied electrical shocks and is not obscured by pacing stimuli artifact. Although it has been restricted mainly to the experimental domain because of voltage dye toxicity, significant strides have been taken toward translation to clinical use. A study carried out recently by Lee and colleagues[50] is notable for development of a fiber-optic mapping method in vivo in an open chest porcine model. Voltage ratiometry (to diminish motion artifact) was carried out using near-infrared voltage dyes (to minimize spectral crosstalk) to examine activation patterns during induced ventricular fibrillation and cardiac pacing. Near-infrared dyes exhibit optimal excitation spectra in the myocardium and are further removed from the maximum excitation wavelength of native chromophores, such as hemoglobin.[51,52] The ultimate milestone would be development of an all-optical electrophysiologic system and is an exciting prospect to look forward to.

Artificial intelligence and machine learning constitute another area in medicine that is progressing at a rapid pace. In the arena of cardiac mapping, it has been implemented commercially in the Ablacon platform, which currently awaits

Food and Drug Administration approval. This system measures endocardial unipolar voltage data using a 64-electrode basket catheter and derives an electrographic flow map in the space and time domains.[53] Overall, innovations in HD mapping and novel multielectrode catheter designs are anticipated to gradually uncloak the entire 3D cardiac architecture and also incorporate highly intelligent systems with machine learning capabilities.

SUMMARY

Cardiac mapping has evolved from the era of sequential PBP mapping to the current paradigm of HD mapping with novel multielectrode catheters. Compared with PBP mapping, HD mapping presents opportunities to enhance AF substrate delineation, greatly improve the efficiency of the mapping procedure without compromising safety, and afford new mechanistic insights regarding AF. We look to the future to bring further refinements in automated HD mapping including evolution of noncontact methodologies and artificial intelligence to supplant current techniques.

DISCLOSURE

Dr P. Santangeli is a consultant for Abbott and Biosense Webster.

REFERENCES

1. Haissaguerre M, Jais P, Shah DC, et al. Spontaneous initiation of atrial fibrillation by ectopic beats originating in the pulmonary veins. N Engl J Med 1998;339:659–66.
2. Lin WS, Tai CT, Hsieh MH, et al. Catheter ablation of paroxysmal atrial fibrillation initiated by nonpulmonary vein ectopy. Circulation 2003;107: 3176–83.
3. Lee SH, Tai CT, Hsieh MH, et al. Predictors of nonpulmonary vein ectopic beats initiating paroxysmal atrial fibrillation: implication for catheter ablation. J Am Coll Cardiol 2005;46:1054–9.
4. Santangeli P, Zado ES, Hutchinson MD, et al. Prevalence and distribution of focal triggers in persistent and long-standing persistent atrial fibrillation. Heart Rhythm 2016;13:374–82.
5. Bhargava M, Di Biase L, Mohanty P, et al. Impact of type of atrial fibrillation and repeat catheter ablation on long-term freedom from atrial fibrillation: results from a multicenter study. Heart Rhythm 2009;6: 1403–12.
6. Tzou Wendy S, Marchlinski Francis E, Zado Erica S, et al. Long-term outcome after successful catheter ablation of atrial fibrillation. Circ Arrhythm Electrophysiol 2010;3:237–42.
7. Kapa S, Desjardins B, Callans DJ, et al. Contact electroanatomic mapping derived voltage criteria for characterizing left atrial scar in patients undergoing ablation for atrial fibrillation. J Cardiovasc Electrophysiol 2014;25:1044–52.
8. Pashakhanloo F, Herzka DA, Ashikaga H, et al. Myofiber architecture of the human atria as revealed by submillimeter diffusion tensor imaging. Circ Arrhythm Electrophysiol 2016;9:e004133.
9. Groot ND, Does LVD, Yaksh A, et al. Direct proof of endo-epicardial asynchrony of the atrial wall during atrial fibrillation in humans. Circ Arrhythm Electrophysiol 2016;9:e003648.
10. Spach MS, Dolber PC. Relating extracellular potentials and their derivatives to anisotropic propagation at a microscopic level in human cardiac muscle. Evidence for electrical uncoupling of side-to-side fiber connections with increasing age. Circ Res 1986;58: 356–71.
11. Spach MS, Miller WT 3rd, Miller-Jones E, et al. Extracellular potentials related to intracellular action potentials during impulse conduction in anisotropic canine cardiac muscle. Circ Res 1979;45:188–204.
12. Stevenson WG, Soejima K. Recording techniques for clinical electrophysiology. J Cardiovasc Electrophysiol 2005;16:1017–22.
13. de Bakker JM, Wittkampf FH. The pathophysiologic basis of fractionated and complex electrograms and the impact of recording techniques on their detection and interpretation. Circ Arrhythm Electrophysiol 2010;3:204–13.
14. Ndrepepa G, Caref EB, Yin H, et al. Activation time determination by high-resolution unipolar and bipolar extracellular electrograms in the canine heart. J Cardiovasc Electrophysiol 1995;6:174–88.
15. Williams SE, Linton NWF, Harrison J, et al. Intra-atrial conduction delay revealed by multisite incremental atrial pacing is an independent marker of remodeling in human atrial fibrillation. JACC Clin Electrophysiol 2017;3:1006–17.
16. Wong GR, Nalliah CJ, Lee G, et al. Dynamic atrial substrate during high-density mapping of paroxysmal and persistent AF: implications for substrate ablation. JACC Clin Electrophysiol 2019;5(11): 1265–77.
17. Sim I, Bishop M, O'Neill M, et al. Left atrial voltage mapping: defining and targeting the atrial fibrillation substrate. J Interv Card Electrophysiol 2019;56(3): 213–27.
18. Tung R, Josephson ME, Bradfield JS, et al. Directional influences of ventricular activation on myocardial scar characterization: voltage mapping with multiple wavefronts during ventricular tachycardia ablation. Circ Arrhythm Electrophysiol 2016;9 [pii: e004155].
19. Liuba I, Walfridsson H. Activation mapping of focal atrial tachycardia: the impact of the method for

estimating activation time. J Interv Card Electrophysiol 2009;26:169–80.

20. Anter E, Tschabrunn CM, Josephson ME. High-resolution mapping of scar-related atrial arrhythmias using smaller electrodes with closer interelectrode spacing. Circ Arrhythm Electrophysiol 2015;8:537–45.

21. Beheshti M, Magtibay K, Massé S, et al. Determinants of atrial bipolar voltage: inter electrode distance and wavefront angle. Comput Biol Med 2018;102:449–57.

22. Takigawa M, Relan J, Martin R, et al. Detailed analysis of the relation between bipolar electrode spacing and far- and near-field electrograms. JACC Clin Electrophysiol 2019;5:66–77.

23. Ndrepepa G, Schneider MA, Karch MR, et al. Impact of atrial fibrillation on the voltage of bipolar signals acquired from the left and right atria. Pacing Clin Electrophysiol 2003;26:862–9.

24. Sasaki N, Watanabe I, Okumura Y, et al. Complex fractionated atrial electrograms, high dominant frequency regions, and left atrial voltages during sinus rhythm and atrial fibrillation. J Arrhythm 2017;33:185–91.

25. Jadidi AS, Duncan E, Miyazaki S, et al. Functional nature of electrogram fractionation demonstrated by left atrial high-density mapping. Circ Arrhythm Electrophysiol 2012;5:32–42.

26. Rodriguez-Manero M, Valderrabano M, Baluja A, et al. Validating left atrial low voltage areas during atrial fibrillation and atrial flutter using multielectrode automated electroanatomic mapping. JACC Clin Electrophysiol 2018;4:1541–52.

27. Yagishita A, Sparano D, Cakulev I, et al. Identification and electrophysiological characterization of early left atrial structural remodeling as a predictor for atrial fibrillation recurrence after pulmonary vein isolation. J Cardiovasc Electrophysiol 2017;28:642–50.

28. Deno DC, Balachandran R, Morgan D, et al. Orientation-independent catheter-based characterization of myocardial activation. IEEE Trans Biomed Eng 2017;64:1067–77.

29. Masse S, Magtibay K, Jackson N, et al. Resolving myocardial activation with novel omnipolar electrograms. Circ Arrhythm Electrophysiol 2016;9:e004107.

30. Magtibay K, Massé S, Asta J, et al. Abstract 17771: novel ventricular voltage mapping methodology with omnipolar electrograms. Circulation 2016;134:A17771.

31. Haldar SK, Magtibay K, Porta-Sanchez A, et al. Resolving bipolar electrogram voltages during atrial fibrillation using omnipolar mapping. Circ Arrhythm Electrophysiol 2017;10:e005018.

32. Linton NW, Koa-Wing M, Francis DP, et al. Cardiac ripple mapping: a novel three-dimensional visualization method for use with electroanatomic mapping of cardiac arrhythmias. Heart rhythm 2009;6:1754–62.

33. Anter E, Duytschaever M, Shen C, et al. Activation mapping with integration of vector and velocity information improves the ability to identify the mechanism and location of complex scar-related atrial tachycardias. Circ Arrhythm Electrophysiol 2018;11:e006536.

34. Sroubek J, Rottmann M, Barkagan M, et al. A novel octaray multielectrode catheter for high-resolution atrial mapping: electrogram characterization and utility for mapping ablation gaps. J Cardiovasc Electrophysiol 2019;30:749–57.

35. van Oosterom A. Solidifying the solid angle. J Electrocardiol 2002;35(Suppl):181–92.

36. Grace A, Willems S, Meyer C, et al. High-resolution noncontact charge-density mapping of endocardial activation. JCI Insight 2019;4:e126422.

37. Willems S, Verma A, Betts TR, et al. Targeting non-pulmonary vein sources in persistent atrial fibrillation identified by noncontact charge density mapping. Circ Arrhythm Electrophysiol 2019;12:e007233.

38. Verma A, Wazni OM, Marrouche NF, et al. Pre-existent left atrial scarring in patients undergoing pulmonary vein antrum isolation: an independent predictor of procedural failure. J Am Coll Cardiol 2005;45:285–92.

39. Marrouche NF, Wilber D, Hindricks G, et al. Association of atrial tissue fibrosis identified by delayed enhancement MRI and atrial fibrillation catheter ablation: the DECAAF study. Jama 2014;311:498–506.

40. Teh AW, Kistler PM, Lee G, et al. Electroanatomic remodeling of the left atrium in paroxysmal and persistent atrial fibrillation patients without structural heart disease. J Cardiovasc Electrophysiol 2012;23:232–8.

41. Garcia-Bolao I, Ballesteros G, Ramos P, et al. Identification of pulmonary vein reconnection gaps with high-density mapping in redo atrial fibrillation ablation procedures. Europace 2018;20:f351–8.

42. Segerson NM, Lynch B, Mozes J, et al. High-density mapping and ablation of concealed low-voltage activity within pulmonary vein antra results in improved freedom from atrial fibrillation compared to pulmonary vein isolation alone. Heart Rhythm 2018;15:1158–64.

43. Rottner L, Metzner A, Ouyang F, et al. Direct comparison of point-by-point and rapid ultra-high-resolution electroanatomical mapping in patients scheduled for ablation of atrial fibrillation. J Cardiovasc Electrophysiol 2017;28:289–97.

44. Hindricks G, Weiner S, McElderry T, et al. Acute safety, effectiveness, and real-world clinical usage of ultra-high density mapping for ablation of cardiac

arrhythmias: results of the TRUE HD study. Europace 2019;21:655–61.

45. Hernandez-Madrid A, Paul T, Abrams D, et al. Arrhythmias in congenital heart disease: a position paper of the European Heart Rhythm Association (EHRA), Association for European Paediatric and Congenital Cardiology (AEPC), and the European Society of Cardiology (ESC) Working Group on Grown-up Congenital heart disease, endorsed by HRS, PACES, APHRS, and SOLAECE. Europace 2018;20:1719–53.

46. Alken F-A, Klatt N, Muenkler P, et al. Advanced mapping strategies for ablation therapy in adults with congenital heart disease. Cardiovasc Diagn Ther 2019;9:S247–63.

47. Mantziari L, Butcher C, Shi R, et al. Characterization of the mechanism and substrate of atrial tachycardia using ultra high density mapping in adults with congenital heart disease: impact on clinical outcomes. J Am Heart Assoc 2019;8:e010535.

48. Pathik B, Lee G, Nalliah C, et al. Entrainment and high density three dimensional mapping in right atrial macro-reentry provide critical complementary information: entrainment may unmask "visual reentry" as passive. Heart rhythm 2017;14:1541–9.

49. Herron TJ, Lee P, Jalife J. Optical imaging of voltage and calcium in cardiac cells & tissues. Circ Res 2012;110:609–23.

50. Lee P, Quintanilla JG, Alfonso-Almazán JM, et al. In vivo ratiometric optical mapping enables high-resolution cardiac electrophysiology in pig models. Cardiovasc Res 2019;115:1659–71.

51. Matiukas A, Mitrea BG, Qin M, et al. Near-infrared voltage-sensitive fluorescent dyes optimized for optical mapping in blood-perfused myocardium. Heart rhythm 2007;4:1441–51.

52. Singh-Moon RP, Marboe CC, Hendon CP. Near-infrared spectroscopy integrated catheter for characterization of myocardial tissues: preliminary demonstrations to radiofrequency ablation therapy for atrial fibrillation. Biomed Opt Express 2015;6:2494–511.

53. Swerdlow M, Tamboli M, Alhusseini MI, et al. Comparing phase and electrographic flow mapping for persistent atrial fibrillation. Pacing Clin Electrophysiol 2019;42:499–507.

Advances in Atrial Fibrillation Ablation
Energy Sources Here to Stay

Gurukripa N. Kowlgi, MBBS, MD, Suraj Kapa, MD, FHRS*

KEYWORDS

- Catheter ablation • Atrial fibrillation • Arrhythmia • Thermal energy • Cryoablation • Electroporation

KEY POINTS

- The energy sources used for catheter ablation of atrial fibrillation (AF) ablation have undergone an exceptional journey over the past 50 years.
- Traditional energy sources, such as radiofrequency and cryoablation, have been the mainstay of AF ablation.
- Novel investigations have led to the inclusion of other techniques, such as laser, high-frequency ultrasound, and microwave energy, in the armamentarium of electrophysiologists.
- Despite having access to these modalities, AF has remained one of the most challenging arrhythmias encountered.
- One key issue with the current energy delivery systems is their reliance on thermal energy for creating lesions, introducing the possibility of collateral damage.

INTRODUCTION

Atrial fibrillation (AF) is the most prevalent type of cardiac arrhythmia, with upwards of 30 million people affected worldwide.[1] The past 3 decades have witnessed a meteoric rise in the treatment options available for AF, and catheter ablation has emerged as a first-line therapy for symptomatic AF.[2,3] What started as simple box diagrams on a Saturday afternoon by Dr James Cox[4–6] has now grown in leaps and bounds, with the various iterations of the Cox-maze procedure. The Maze procedure provided the electrophysiologic construct of pulmonary vein isolation (PVI), which has been expanded on by many pioneering electrophysiologists.[7–9]

The backbone of AF ablation is the ability to create durable lines of conduction block within the atria. Although the classic cut-and-sew surgical approaches of AF ablation revolutionized the field, they demanded sternotomies, cardiopulmonary bypass, and long procedures as well as recovery durations. Developments in the field have thus converged on adopting minimally invasive techniques that are quicker and safer and deliver effective lesions while minimizing collateral damage.[10]

The success of catheter-based AF ablation, even at experienced centers, is approximately 70%, although with a wide standard deviation in outcomes.[11] Nontransmural lesions at sites of ablation have been reported as a frequent cause of AF recurrences.[12,13] The pursuit of the ideal energy source has led to a multitude of choices for the modern-day electrophysiologist. The goal of this review is to educate readers regarding the advances in the various sources of energy that can be used for AF ablation.

RADIOFREQUENCY ABLATION
Background and Biophysics

The formative years of catheter ablation witnessed the use of direct current and chemical energy for ablation. The advent of radiofrequency ablation

Department of Cardiovascular Medicine, Mayo Clinic, 200 First Street Southwest, Rochester, MN 55905, USA
* Corresponding author.
E-mail address: kapa.suraj@mayo.edu

Card Electrophysiol Clin 12 (2020) 167–174
https://doi.org/10.1016/j.ccep.2020.02.005
1877-9182/20/© 2020 Elsevier Inc. All rights reserved.

(RFA) was a substantial advance in the field, and, currently, RFA is the preferred energy source in most electrophysiology laboratories around the world.[14] The radiofrequency (RF) band employs frequencies between 30 kHz to 30,000 kHz for ablation, with 550 kHz the most common operating frequency.[15,16] RF energy is delivered via alternating current through a small probe, which increases current density. The current travels from the platinum-iridium electrode tip through the body toward a dispersive grounding pad attached at the back. The mode of tissue destruction is thermal, more specifically, resistive heating, which refers to direct heating of a thin rim of adjacent tissue up to 1 mm deep. Deeper layers are not heated directly due to the phenomenon of energy dissipation with distance.[17] The mechanism of deep tissue heating is passive conductive heating from the superficial layers.[18] Conductive heating has a greater impact on lesion volume than resistive heating.

Clinical correlate

Contact force (CF) and duration are vital cogs in RFA. Force results in effective resistive heating, and duration is responsible for heating deeper layers via conductive heating. In practice, 10 g to 20 g of force over 60 seconds to 120 seconds creates effective lesions.[19,20]

Cellular Changes During Ablation

Myocardial tissue suffers irreversible damage at temperatures beyond 50°C, with resultant coagulation and destruction of cellular structures. In the acute phase, the ability of the cell to sequester calcium is disrupted due to the impairment of the sarcoplasmic reticulum.[21] Energy dissipation occurs due to convective effects of blood at the endocardial surface as well as blood vessels in the epicardium that can act as heat sinks.[16,22,23] Over time, this tissue is replaced by collagen scar and fibrin. If the cellular temperature reaches 45°C to 50°C, the damage can be reversible and give rise to reconnections after acutely successful ablation.[16]

Clinical correlate

With nonirrigated catheters, when peak electrode-tissue contact temperature of 100°C is reached, serum proteins are denatured and adhere to the electrode tip, forming an insulating coating. If this is observed, power output should be decreased rapidly to avoid sudden rises in impedance, charring, tissue adherence, and even thrombus formation.

Lesion Size Determinants

Multiple factors can affect lesion size with RFA. Greater CF, longer duration, higher power, and electrode temperature all lead to deeper lesions. Larger electrodes with larger source diameter can increase lesion size proportionally. Higher power increases lesion size both by increasing the diameter of the heat source and by elevating the source temperature. Unipolar ablation is well controlled, but lesions can take a long time to develop.[10] To produce lesions 3 mm to 6 mm deep, it takes application of RF at 80°C for 1 minute.[24] The operator must observe caution because the maximum tissue temperature does not occur at the point of contact with the catheter. Instead, it occurs just below the contact surface, which renders the risk of thermal injury to adjacent structures, especially in thin-walled structures.[25] Convective cooling and tissue resistance can serve as barriers to effective ablation.[23]

CF science has been revisited in the past 5 years with the emergence of CF sensing catheters. Although early nonrandomized data were promising,[26] subsequent randomized trials have not reproduced improvement in clinical endpoints.[27] The general consensus now is that although CF is a critical factor in determining lesion size, quality with regard to catheter contact should be the objective. Quality considers spatiotemporal dynamics, such as catheter stability, catheter drift, and cardiac and respiratory motion gating.[28]

Finally, to tackle the challenge of reaching effective tissue temperatures without causing impedance rise and char formation, irrigated catheter systems were invented and are the norm today for RFA, particularly for AF.[29] With irrigated ablation, the effects of resistive heating can be delivered 3 mm to 4 mm below the contact surface. With irrigated catheters, however, the electrode tip temperature is not an ideal determinant of lesion formation.[30] Conventional settings for irrigated catheters include 25-W, 50-mL/min saline irrigation with lesions of 4-mm to 5-mm depth able to be created within 20 seconds.[31]

Clinical correlate

Caution must be exercised, especially while using irrigated catheters, when it comes to estimating tissue temperature. When temperatures exceed 100°C, intramyocardial steam develops and can result in steam pops, which can dissect along muscle planes and result in tamponade or perforation.[30]

Updates in Radiofrequency Technology

Owing to long procedure times with conventional point-by-point RFA, circular catheters with multiple electrodes were developed, which simultaneously could create long contiguous lesion sets.[32] These catheters also were equipped with duty cycle phasing, which allowed alternating be-tween unipolar and bipolar energy delivery. Although lower fluoroscopy times were noted,[33] there were concerns raised about greater risk of asymptomatic cerebral embolization with the use of nonirrigated multielectrode catheters.[34] Further refinement in catheter technology has led to the creation of a catheter with a diamond-embedded tip for surface cooling and 6 thermocouples that can accomplish temperature-controlled irrigated RFA for PVI.[35] These catheter systems can achieve dynamic power modulation based on con-tact and accurate tip temperatures for safe and effective lesions. A discussion of RFA is incom-plete without mention of recent strategies that challenge the conventional relationship of resistive and conductive heating. High-power short-dura-tion ablation (90 W/4 s) is one such technique that creates wider lesions that are consistently transmural.[36,37] High-power short-duration can be an enticing option for AF ablation, but accurate temperature measuring electrodes would be paramount.

Advantages/Disadvantages

RFA is a simple and effective method of creating continuous and transmural ablations. It has been tried and tested over years of clinical use.[38] There is an assortment of different catheter shapes and designs suited for variations in anatomy and oper-ator preference.

The disadvantages of using RFA relate to ther-mal latency and the lack of tissue specificity. Because conductive heating determines a majority of the lesion volume, tissue temperatures continue to rise even after ablation is terminated. Thermal injury can lead to the destruction of adjacent tis-sue. The list of potential complications includes pulmonary vein (PV) stenosis, atrioesophageal fis-tula, and phrenic nerve injury.[39] RFA is regarded as the most thrombogenic energy source. As a result of inadvertent char formation, RFA can cause intracavitary thrombus and possibly stroke; hence, astute observation and vigilance during RFA cannot be overstated.

CRYOABLATION
Background and Biophysics

Cryoablation produces myocardial tissue necrosis utilizing extreme cooling. The original application of cryoablation was in the 1980s in surgical epicar-dial accessory pathway ablation.[40] Cryoablation received approval from the Food and Drug Admin-istration before RFA for cardiac arrhythmias. It was not until 2007, however, that cryoballoon technol-ogy was described for AF ablation in a feasibility study[41] and subsequently supported by random-ized controlled trials.[42]

Commercially available cryoballoon catheters have an inner balloon, where the refrigerant liquid nitrous oxide gets delivered and undergoes a phase change to produced cooling via the Joule-Thomson effect. This process results in tempera-ture drop to almost −80°C, which is monitored by a thermocouple located at the inner balloon. The catheter has a spiral mapping catheter that projects through a central lumen. The spiral cath-eter decreases perforation risk by guiding the balloon catheter safely into PVs and serves the purpose of mapping PV potentials.

Clinical correlate
Similar to RFA, contact is essential for cryoabla-tion. Imaging modalities, such as intracardiac echocardiography with color flow Doppler, frequently are used to confirm cryoballoon contact at the PV ostium.

Cellular Changes During Ablation

The primary mechanism of lesion formation in cry-oablation is direct cellular injury. Cryoablation pro-duces tissue destruction in phases. In the initial freeze-thaw phase, the cold temperature at the catheter tip draws heat out of healthy tissue, lead-ing to the formation of extracellular and intracel-lular ice crystals. The crystals cause compression and osmotic distortion of cell mem-branes and intracellular organelles within a few hours, leading to irreversible lesions. At approxi-mately 48 hours, inflammation and hemorrhage ensue in phase 2, leading to more cellular destruc-tion via edema and apoptosis. Finally, phase 3 is composed of tissue infiltration by inflammatory cells and eventual fibrosis over weeks.[43] As a sup-plement to direct cellular injury, cryoablation also produces vascular injury that enhances lesion for-mation. Vascular injury is initiated by vasoconstric-tion, and with subfreezing temperatures, endothelial damage and microthrombotic occlu-sions are responsible for ischemic necrosis.[44]

Clinical correlate
Extracellular ice formation and apoptosis take a few minutes to develop a window of reversibility with cryoablation lesions, which is why cryoabla-tion often is designated the forgiving energy source.

Lesion Size Determinants

Lower catheter temperatures lead to larger le-sions, as expected. The other factors that increase lesion size include rapid cooling, longer duration of freezing, and a higher number of cycles. The utilization of free-thaw-refreeze cycles seems to increase lesion durability as well.[45] As with RFA, catheter contact is a critical ingredient for successful cryoablation.

Clinical correlate

One notable difference in cryoablation compared with RFA is the uncomplicated relation to distance and tissue injury. The coldest site is intuitively the tissue in contact with the catheter. Distant sites can be affected but often in a reversible fashion. Latent injury in sites not directly in contact with the catheter can happen, albeit rarely.

Updates in Cryoablation Technology

One practical technique that has been described with cryoablation is cryomapping. This method allows cooling myocardial tissue to −30°C, such that irreversible damage is avoided. With the application of cryomapping, the operator can observe for brief physiologic changes. If these changes include collateral damage, such as phrenic nerve injury or coronary artery damage, a full-fledged lesion is not delivered.

Second-generation cryoballoon catheters are equipped with multiple nitrous oxide jets, which cool the distal half of the balloon.[46] Although the efficacy may be improved from the first-generation described in the STOP-AF (Sustained Treatment of Paroxysmal Atrial Fibrillation) trial,[42] predilections for damage of surrounding structures may be higher. The FIRE AND ICE (Cryoballoon or Radiofrequency Ablation for Paroxysmal Atrial Fibrillation) trial deemed both generations of cryoablation catheters as noninferior to RFA in drug-refractory paroxysmal AF patients.[47] Recent registry data suggest that cryoablation may be superior to RFA for AF due to lower reablation rates, although this has not been corroborated by head-to-head trials.[48]

Advantages/Disadvantages

One major advantage of using cryoablation in contrast to RFA is the ability to preserve collagen and, thus, maintain tissue architecture. There exists a window of reversibility, which makes it possible to avoid serious complications if cryoenergy is turned off. Cryomapping, as elucidated previously, is a suitable adjunct. A vital feature of cryoablation is the stability of contact rendered by ice formation, which results in consistent tissue injury. Shorter procedure times are another big strategic plus with cryoablation.

Cryoablation has been shown to result in a higher percentage of phrenic nerve palsy. Although a majority of phrenic nerve injury resolve within a year, a small proportion may persist permanently.[47]

Clinical correlate

Cryoablation catheters are stiffer than RFA catheters and must be handled with caution to avoid PV perforation and inadvertent damage to surrounding structures.

MISCELLANEOUS SOURCES OF ENERGY
Laser Ablation

Lasers have an optical coupling fiber and a radiating fiber tip that produce high-energy coherent beams. Modern laser ablation catheters utilize 980-nm wavelength diode laser, which is absorbed primarily by the water in the tissue resulting in dielectric heating. In addition to direct heating, the tissue also suffers mechanical damage caused by shock waves. Reddy and colleagues[49] described the feasibility of a variable-diameter compliant balloon with simultaneous endoscopic visualization of the PVs and diode laser for ablation. The investigators noted that the efficacy of laser catheter ablation was good, but adverse events included cardiac tamponade, phrenic nerve injury, and stroke. Subsequent, randomized controlled trials demonstrated noninferiority of laser balloon ablation compared with RFA in paroxysmal AF.

The advantages of laser balloon catheters include stable position and contiguous lesions with the added ability to titrate energy at different areas on the circumferential lesion set. The diameter of the balloon is flexible, which allows access despite variations in PV anatomy. In the surgical literature, one of the disadvantages of laser ablation was the lack of a safety mechanism at high temperatures, akin to char formation in RFA. As a result, high energy can cause crater formation and even tissue perforation.[50]

High-Intensity Focused Ultrasound

High-intensity focused ultrasound (HIFU) in the range of 20 kHz to 200 MHz produces tissue destruction by localized hyperthermic lesions. Ultrasound waves passing through tissue, causing oscillation in water molecules. The kinetic energy generated as a result is converted to thermal injury. As a direct consequence, if the source power is too high, it may lead to excess tissue shearing and damage to collateral structures. Although CF is not a prerequisite for ablation, the inability to control segmental circumferential energy can produce unwanted outcomes. A safety algorithm was developed by Neven and colleagues[51] for HIFU-based PVI, which was unsuccessful in preventing complications, such as phrenic nerve palsy and atrioesophageal fistula. Human trials using HIFU catheter-based ablation were suspended based on these adverse events. HIFU may still offer promise in surgical epicardial ablation, where it has been demonstrated that transmural lesions are possible and unimpeded by epicardial fat.[52]

Microwave Ablation

Similar to laser and HIFU, microwaves can cause oscillation of water molecules in the myocardium, resulting in dielectric heating without char formation. Microwave energy produces radiant heating; hence, noncontact ablation is a possibility. Microwaves can have some tissue selectivity owing to differences in water content, such that it penetrates through low-water content tissue, such as fat, and get absorbed in relatively higher water–content myocardium, producing heat. Promising results have been seen in an in vitro model of PV antrum.[53]

PULSED FIELD ABLATION
Background and Biophysics

The application of a strong, pulsed electric field can cause increased permeability of the cell membrane (pore formation), leading to irreversible electroporation. This modality has been utilized for tumor ablation for many years.[54] The enthusiasm surrounding pulsed field ablation (PFA) has to do with its nonthermal mode of cellular injury, the reported tissue specificity, and the relatively rapid energy deliver compared with conventional sources. The electric field is usually generated by high-voltage direct current between 2 or more electrodes. The electric field establishes charge across the lipid bilayer. Depending on transmembrane voltage, irreversible electroporation occurs when a critical threshold of charge is reached. Most PEF protocols use ultrashort pulses lasting nanoseconds, at low frequency, to prevent any heat generated due to resistance.[55] Hence, electroporation can be considered a nonthermal source of energy if applied with the techniques, described previously.

Preclinical studies on PFA have demonstrated the safety and efficacy of direct current ablation when applied to the PV antrum in AF.[56–58] The lower risk of collateral damage to nontarget tissue was a recurrent theme with PFA studies.[59,60] Direct comparison of PFA and RF demonstrated a lower incidence of PV stenosis with PFA.[61] The solitary in-human study of PFA was conducted by Reddy and colleagues[62] in patients with paroxysmal AF. In this study, a custom generator was used to deliver high-voltage pulsed field energy through multiple channels. Two different kinds of catheters were used with endocardial and epicardial approaches, respectively, through a steerable 13F sheath. Flexible programming was built in with various waveforms and bipolar electrode-pairing options. Investigators in this study described that PFA could be used to selectively affect myocardial tissues safely and effectively while minimizing collateral damage.

Cellular Changes During Ablation

After the application of PFA, microscopic pores at approximately 10 nm in size form within nanoseconds.[63] Water molecules, driven by local transmembrane gradients, penetrate the cell membrane hastening pore formation.[64] Multiple studies have shown that deep lesions (more than 1 cm) can be achieved even with a single high-voltage application of PFA. Although some of the investigators have demonstrated that electroporation can cause inflammation and myocardial fiber disruption but no coagulation necrosis,[65] others have described chronic inflammation, fibroblast proliferation, and scar formation in lesions.[66] The histologic descriptions of PFA have been quite variable across studies.

Clinical correlate
The relative differences in resting membrane potential change the threshold for tissue damage, conferring an inherent tissue selectivity to PFA. This feature minimizes damage to noncardiac structures.

Factors Affecting Lesion Size

The tissue effects of PFA depends on certain characteristics of the applied electric field: voltage, frequency, polarity, and pulse duration. One key finding of electroporation studies is the graded effect from reversible damage to irreversible apoptosis, depending on the intensity of the applied electric field. Low energy can cause reversible pore formation, which has been useful in drug delivery systems, but higher energy can lead to irreversible electroporation, apoptosis, and cell death.

Clinical correlate
Since PFA theoretically has more tissue selectivity, the possibility of forming reversible lesions may not have as much of a practical impact as we see with cryomapping. However, this may minimize ablations performed on healthy myocardium.

Advantages/Disadvantages

With the present level of understanding of PFA, there seem to be many favorable attributes that make it potentially useful. The reported benefits of PFA over the traditional sources of energy include tissue selectivity and the potential for ultra-rapid PV isolation. Notwithstanding all these positive traits of PFA, like any new technology, caution must be exercised for what may not yet be known. Specifically, these would include the lack of clinical data with longer-term follow-up in humans to assess for late complications; equipment issues, such as the widespread availability of a dedicated cardiac generator system; and technical factors, with the ability to titrate energy fields by providers, making standardization across health systems a herculean task.

SUMMARY

Despite decades of work by some fantastic minds, AF has remained an elusive target. Does the answer lie in a better understanding of the pathophysiology, or does it have to do with the imperfect ways of ablating a known target? There is a whole gamut of options available in the arsenal of the modern electrophysiologist when dealing with AF ablation. Although there are many promising avenues, further investigations are needed to refine the existing energy sources and determine if any one provides the optimal path to long-term success.

REFERENCES

1. Chugh SS, Havmoeller R, Narayanan K, et al. Worldwide epidemiology of atrial fibrillation. Circulation 2014;129(8):837–47.
2. January CT, Wann LS, Alpert JS, et al. 2014 AHA/ACC/HRS guideline for the management of patients with atrial fibrillation. J Am Coll Cardiol 2014;64(21):e1–76.
3. Calkins H, Reynolds MR, Spector P, et al. Treatment of atrial fibrillation with antiarrhythmic drugs or radiofrequency ablation. Circ Arrhythm Electrophysiol 2009;2(4):349–61.
4. Cox JL. HRS 40th anniversary viewpoints: reflections on a career in arrhythmia surgery. Heart Rhythm 2019;16(4):638–9.
5. Cox JL, Schuessler RB, Boineau JP. The surgical treatment of atrial fibrillation. I. Summary of the current concepts of the mechanisms of atrial flutter and atrial fibrillation. J Thorac Cardiovasc Surg 1991;101(3):402–5.
6. Cox JL, Canavan TE, Schuessler RB, et al. The surgical treatment of atrial fibrillation. II. Intraoperative electrophysiologic mapping and description of the electrophysiologic basis of atrial flutter and atrial fibrillation. J Thorac Cardiovasc Surg 1991;101(3):406–26.
7. Haïssaguerre M, Jaïs P, Shah DC, et al. Spontaneous initiation of atrial fibrillation by ectopic beats originating in the pulmonary veins. N Engl J Med 1998;339(10):659–66.
8. Maloney JD, Milner L, Barold S, et al. Two-staged biatrial linear and focal ablation to restore sinus rhythm in patients with refractory chronic atrial fibrillation: procedure experience and follow-up beyond 1 year. Pacing Clin Electrophysiol 1998;21(11):2527–32.
9. Manolis AS, Wang PJ, Estes NA. Radiofrequency catheter ablation for cardiac tachyarrhythmias. Ann Intern Med 1994;121(6):452.
10. Comas GM, Imren Y, Williams MR. An overview of energy sources in clinical use for the ablation of atrial fibrillation. Semin Thorac Cardiovasc Surg 2007;19(1):16–24.
11. Cappato R, Calkins H, Chen S-A, et al. Updated worldwide survey on the methods, efficacy, and safety of catheter ablation for human atrial fibrillation. Circ Arrhythm Electrophysiol 2010;3(1):32–8.
12. Kowalski M, Grimes MM, Perez FJ, et al. Histopathologic characterization of chronic radiofrequency ablation lesions for pulmonary vein isolation. J Am Coll Cardiol 2012;59(10):930–8.
13. Nanthakumar K, Plumb VJ, Epstein AE, et al. Resumption of electrical conduction in previously isolated pulmonary veins. Circulation 2004;109(10):1226–9.
14. Ouyang F, Tilz R, Chun J, et al. Long-term results of catheter ablation in paroxysmal atrial fibrillation. Circulation 2010;122(23):2368–77.
15. Arora PK, Hansen JC, Price AD, et al. An update on the energy sources and catheter technology for the ablation of atrial fibrillation. J Atr Fibrillation 2010;2(5):233.
16. Haines DE. The biophysics of radiofrequency catheter ablation in the heart: the importance of temperature monitoring. Pacing Clin Electrophysiol 1993;16(3 Pt 2):586–91.
17. Strohbehn JW. Temperature distributions from interstitial RF electrode hyperthermia systems: theoretical predictions. Int J Radiat Oncol Biol Phys 1983;9(11):1655–67.
18. Haines DE, Watson DD. Tissue heating during radiofrequency catheter ablation: a thermodynamic model and observations in isolated perfused and superfused canine right ventricular free wall. Pacing Clin Electrophysiol 1989;12(6):962–76.
19. Gaita F, Riccardi R, Calò L, et al. Atrial mapping and radiofrequency catheter ablation in patients with idiopathic atrial fibrillation. Electrophysiological findings and ablation results. Circulation 1998;97(21):2136–45.

20. Williams SE, Harrison J, Chubb H, et al. The effect of contact force in atrial radiofrequency ablation. JACC Clin Electrophysiol 2015;1(5):421–31.

21. Nath S, Lynch C, Whayne JG, et al. Cellular electrophysiological effects of hyperthermia on isolated Guinea pig papillary muscle. Implications for catheter ablation. Circulation 1993;88(4 Pt 1):1826–31.

22. Thomas SP, Nicholson IA, Nunn GR, et al. Effect of atrial radiofrequency ablation designed to cure atrial fibrillation on atrial mechanical function. J Cardiovasc Electrophysiol 2000;11(1):77–82.

23. Raman JS, Seevanayagam S, Storer M, et al. Combined endocardial and epicardial radiofrequency ablation of right and left atria in the treatment of atrial fibrillation. Ann Thorac Surg 2001;72(3):S1096–9.

24. Williams MR, Stewart JR, Bolling SF, et al. Surgical treatment of atrial fibrillation using radiofrequency energy. Ann Thorac Surg 2001;71(6):1939–43.

25. Everett TH, Nath S, Lynch C, et al. Role of calcium in acute hyperthermic myocardial injury. J Cardiovasc Electrophysiol 2001;12(5):563–9.

26. Afzal MR, Chatta J, Samanta A, et al. Use of contact force sensing technology during radiofrequency ablation reduces recurrence of atrial fibrillation: a systematic review and meta-analysis. Heart Rhythm 2015;12(9):1990–6.

27. Ullah W, McLean A, Tayebjee MH, et al. Randomized trial comparing pulmonary vein isolation using the SmartTouch catheter with or without real-time contact force data. Heart Rhythm 2016;13(9):1761–7.

28. Ariyarathna N, Kumar S, Thomas SP, et al. Role of contact force sensing in catheter ablation of cardiac arrhythmias. JACC Clin Electrophysiol 2018;4(6):707–23.

29. Nakagawa H, Yamanashi WS, Pitha JV, et al. Comparison of in vivo tissue temperature profile and lesion geometry for radiofrequency ablation with a saline-irrigated electrode versus temperature control in a canine thigh muscle preparation. Circulation 1995;91(8):2264–73.

30. Wittkampf FHM, Nakagawa H. RF catheter ablation: lessons on lesions. Pacing Clin Electrophysiol 2006;29(11):1285–97.

31. Wong JWW. Ensuring transmurality using irrigated radiofrequency modified maze in surgery for atrial fibrillation—a simple and effective way. Heart Lung Circ 2004;13(3):302–8.

32. Fredersdorf S, Weber S, Jilek C, et al. Safe and rapid isolation of pulmonary veins using a novel circular ablation catheter and duty-cycled RF generator. J Cardiovasc Electrophysiol 2009;20(10):1097–101.

33. Tivig C, Dang L, Brunner-La Rocca H-P, et al. Duty-cycled unipolar/bipolar versus conventional radiofrequency ablation in paroxysmal and persistent atrial fibrillation. Int J Cardiol 2012;157(2):185–91.

34. Herrera Siklódy C, Deneke T, Hocini M, et al. Incidence of asymptomatic intracranial embolic events after pulmonary vein isolation. J Am Coll Cardiol 2011;58(7):681–8.

35. Iwasawa J, Koruth JS, Petru J, et al. Temperature-controlled radiofrequency ablation for pulmonary vein isolation in patients with atrial fibrillation. J Am Coll Cardiol 2017;70(5):542–53.

36. Leshem E, Zilberman I, Tschabrunn CM, et al. High-power and short-duration ablation for pulmonary vein isolation. JACC Clin Electrophysiol 2018;4(4):467–79.

37. Reddy VY, Grimaldi M, De Potter T, et al. Pulmonary vein isolation with very high power, short duration, temperature-controlled lesions. JACC Clin Electrophysiol 2019;5(7):778–86.

38. Nattel S. New ideas about atrial fibrillation 50 years on. Nature 2002;415(6868):219–26.

39. Doll N, Borger MA, Fabricius A, et al. Esophageal perforation during left atrial radiofrequency ablation: is the risk too high? J Thorac Cardiovasc Surg 2003;125(4):836–42.

40. Klein GJ, Guiraudon GM, Perkins DG, et al. Surgical correction of the Wolff-Parkinson-White syndrome in the closed heart using cryosurgery: a simplified approach. J Am Coll Cardiol 1984;3(2 Pt 1):405–9.

41. Van Belle Y, Janse P, Rivero-Ayerza MJ, et al. Pulmonary vein isolation using an occluding cryoballoon for circumferential ablation: feasibility, complications, and short-term outcome. Eur Heart J 2007;28(18):2231–7.

42. Packer DL, Kowal RC, Wheelan KR, et al. Cryoballoon ablation of pulmonary veins for paroxysmal atrial fibrillation. J Am Coll Cardiol 2013;61(16):1713–23.

43. Lustgarten DL, Keane D, Ruskin J. Cryothermal ablation: mechanism of tissue injury and current experience in the treatment of tachyarrhythmias. Prog Cardiovasc Dis 1999;41(6):481–98.

44. Gage AA, Baust J. Mechanisms of tissue injury in cryosurgery. Cryobiology 1998;37(3):171–86.

45. Su W, Aryana A, Passman R, et al. Cryoballoon Best Practices II: practical guide to procedural monitoring and dosing during atrial fibrillation ablation from the perspective of experienced users. Heart Rhythm 2018;15(9):1348–55.

46. Takami M, Misiri J, Lehmann HI, et al. Spatial and time-course thermodynamics during pulmonary vein isolation using the second-generation cryoballoon in a canine in vivo model. Circ Arrhythm Electrophysiol 2015;8(1):186–92.

47. Kuck K-H, Brugada J, Fürnkranz A, et al. Cryoballoon or radiofrequency ablation for paroxysmal atrial fibrillation. N Engl J Med 2016;374(23):2235–45.

48. Mörtsell D, Arbelo E, Dagres N, et al. Cryoballoon vs. radiofrequency ablation for atrial fibrillation: a

study of outcome and safety based on the ESC-EHRA atrial fibrillation ablation long-term registry and the Swedish catheter ablation registry. Europace 2019;21(4):581–9.

49. Reddy VY, Neuzil P, Themistoclakis S, et al. Visually-guided balloon catheter ablation of atrial fibrillation: experimental feasibility and first-in-human multicenter clinical outcome. Circulation 2009;120(1):12–20.

50. Williams MR, Casher JM, Russo MJ, et al. Laser energy source in surgical atrial fibrillation ablation: preclinical experience. Ann Thorac Surg 2006;82(6):2260–4.

51. Neven K, Schmidt B, Metzner A, et al. Fatal end of a safety algorithm for pulmonary vein isolation with use of high-intensity focused ultrasound. Circ Arrhythm Electrophysiol 2010;3(3):260–5.

52. Mitnovetski S, Almeida AA, Goldstein J, et al. Epicardial high-intensity focused ultrasound cardiac ablation for surgical treatment of atrial fibrillation. Heart Lung Circ 2009;18(1):28–31.

53. Qian P, Barry MA, Nguyen T, et al. A novel microwave catheter can perform noncontact circumferential endocardial ablation in a model of pulmonary vein isolation. J Cardiovasc Electrophysiol 2015;26(7):799–804.

54. Martin RCG, McFarland K, Ellis S, et al. Irreversible electroporation in locally advanced pancreatic cancer: potential improved overall survival. Ann Surg Oncol 2013;20(S3):443–9.

55. Davalos RV, Mir LM, Rubinsky B. Tissue ablation with irreversible electroporation. Ann Biomed Eng 2005;33(2):223–31.

56. Wittkampf FH, Van Driel VJ, Van Wessel H, et al. Feasibility of electroporation for the creation of pulmonary vein ostial lesions. J Cardiovasc Electrophysiol 2011;22(3):302–9.

57. DeSimone CV, Ebrille E, Syed FF, et al. Novel balloon catheter device with pacing, ablating, electroporation, and drug-eluting capabilities for atrial fibrillation treatment—preliminary efficacy and safety studies in a canine model. Transl Res 2014;164(6):508–14.

58. Witt CM, Sugrue A, Padmanabhan D, et al. Intrapulmonary vein ablation without stenosis: a novel balloon-based direct current electroporation approach. J Am Heart Assoc 2018;7(14) [pii: e009575].

59. Neven K, van Es R, van Driel V, et al. Acute and long-term effects of full-power electroporation ablation directly on the porcine esophagus. Circ Arrhythm Electrophysiol 2017;10(5) [pii:e004672].

60. van Driel VJHM, Neven K, van Wessel H, et al. Low vulnerability of the right phrenic nerve to electroporation ablation. Heart Rhythm 2015;12(8):1838–44.

61. van Driel VJHM, Neven KGEJ, van Wessel H, et al. Pulmonary vein stenosis after catheter ablation. Circ Arrhythm Electrophysiol 2014;7(4):734–8.

62. Reddy VY, Koruth J, Jais P, et al. Ablation of atrial fibrillation with pulsed electric fields: an ultra-rapid, tissue-selective modality for cardiac ablation. JACC Clin Electrophysiol 2018;4(8):987–95.

63. Tieleman DP. The molecular basis of electroporation. BMC Biochem 2004;5(1):10.

64. Maor E, Sugrue A, Witt C, et al. Pulsed electric fields for cardiac ablation and beyond: a state-of-the-art review. Heart Rhythm 2019;16(7):1112–20.

65. Hong J, Stewart MT, Cheek DS, et al. Cardiac ablation via electroporation. In: 2009 Annual International Conference of the IEEE Engineering in Medicine and Biology Society 3-6 September, 2009: Minneapolis, MN, USA. IEEE; 2009: p. 3381–4.

66. du Pré BC, van Driel VJ, van Wessel H, et al. Minimal coronary artery damage by myocardial electroporation ablation. Europace 2013;15(1):144–9.

Balloon-Based Ablation Technologies

Rahul Bhardwaj, MD[a], Petr Neuzil, MD, PhD[b], Vivek Y. Reddy, MD[c], Srinivas R. Dukkipati, MD[c],*

KEYWORDS

• Atrial fibrillation • Cryoballoon • Laser balloon • Radiofrequency balloon • Pulmonary vein isolation

KEY POINTS

• Balloon-based catheter ablation is an attractive option for the creation of contiguous lesions to achieve pulmonary vein isolation that is less operator dependent.
• Cryoballoon ablation is a well-validated and widely used approach with comparable efficacy and safety to standard radiofrequency ablation and results in comparatively quicker procedures but longer fluoroscopy time.
• Laser balloon is an effective and safe approach to achieve pulmonary vein isolation. Newer iterations of the technology are forthcoming that are under evaluation in clinical trials.
• Several radiofrequency catheter balloons are under evaluation in ongoing clinical trials.

INTRODUCTION

Catheter ablation to achieve pulmonary vein isolation (PVI) is the mainstay of interventional treatment of both persistent and paroxysmal atrial fibrillation.[1] Although additional targets have been implicated, the standard initial approach is antral isolation of all 4 pulmonary veins.[2] Advances in radiofrequency (RF) catheter ablation technology and techniques such as irrigation, force sensing, and utilization of ablation indices to better understand lesion size have improved efficacy, but this approach remains time-consuming and dependent on operator skill. As such, achieving the goal of highly reproducible durable PVI remains elusive because lesions may be ineffective because of lack of transmurality and gaps.[3–5] Ineffective lesions resulting in breakthrough can lead to recurrence of atrial fibrillation or atrial tachycardias. Balloon-based ablation techniques offer a "one-shot" solution to create contiguous lesions to effect PVI that is less dependent on operator dexterity. Several catheter-based balloon ablation devices using varying energy sources are available for clinical use, and new iterations to achieve greater efficacy, efficiency, and safety are in development. In addition, because of the recognition of extrapulmonary vein triggers in persistent atrial fibrillation, such as the left atrial posterior wall, there have been advancements in approaches using existing ablation balloons to effectively treat these areas. This article reviews balloon-based catheter ablation technologies and techniques to treat atrial fibrillation, with a focus on cryoballoon and laser balloon.

CRYOBALLOON

Ablation using cryothermy is well established as a method of treating cardiac arrhythmia and has been used in surgical ablation, endocardial focal

[a] Loma Linda University, 11234 Anderson Street, Suite 1636, Loma Linda, CA 92354, USA; [b] Na Homolce Hospital, Roentgenova 2, 15030 Prague, Czech Republic; [c] Helmsley Electrophysiology Center, Icahn School of Medicine at Mount Sinai, One Gustave L. Levy Place, Box 1030, New York, New York 10029, USA
* Corresponding author.
E-mail address: Srinivas.dukkipati@mountsinai.org

Card Electrophysiol Clin 12 (2020) 175–185
https://doi.org/10.1016/j.ccep.2020.02.008
1877-9182/20/© 2020 Elsevier Inc. All rights reserved.

ablation, and balloon-based ablation. An advantage of cryoablation is that when used, the act of freezing will cause the catheter to adhere to tissue and consequently improve stability. Tissue cooling initially reversibly damages myocardium, and with longer lesions or colder temperature, irreversibly ablates tissue. Cryoablation injures myocardial tissue by the 3 following methods: (1) the freezing and thawing process, (2) hemorrhage and inflammation, and (3) fibrosis and apoptosis.[6]

Technology and Technique

Cryoballoon catheters currently clinically available in the United States include the Arctic Front Cryoballoon (Medtronic, Inc, Minneapolis, MN, USA) and its successors: the second-generation Arctic Front Advance and third-generation Arctic Front Advance Pro. The balloon is composed of an outer polyurethane balloon and inner polyester balloon that attach to a 10.5F shaft with pull wires, a thermocouple, and a guidewire lumen. The devices are offered with a fixed 23-mm or 28-mm diameter. The catheter system is advanced through a 12F steerable sheath into the left atrium over a wire or mapping catheter under fluoroscopic and intracardiac echocardiography (ICE) guidance. The transseptal puncture is optimally low and mid to anterior on the septum to facilitate optimal balloon positioning. Before insertion, the balloon is prepared in a saline bath to ensure all air is removed from the system. The balloon may be advanced over a wire or over a dedicated multielectrode spiral mapping catheter (Achieve; Medtronic, Inc), which guides positioning of the balloon and can record pulmonary vein potentials during and after ablation. After positioning the balloon at the ostium of the target vein, it is inflated and pressure is applied to occlude the vein and thus ensure circumferential contact of the balloon to the atrial tissue. Contrast injected through the shaft of the catheter informs the operator about effectiveness of the catheter occlusion of the vein. Once adequate position and contact are achieved, the cryoablation system is activated, and liquid N_2O is injected into the inner balloon from an injector tube in the shaft and can reach temperatures of $-80^{\circ}C$. The second-generation device improved on the first-generation cryoballoon with improvement in coolant delivery by increasing the number of refrigerant jets from 4 to 8 in the balloon and positioning the jets more distally, resulting in more distal and uniform cooling. This improvement has resulted in greater efficiency and efficacy in PVI.[7,8] As clinical experience with the cryoballoon has increased, there has been recognition of

particular factors that can result in greater efficacy, such as time to isolation (TTI).[9] TTI is sometimes difficult to appreciate because the mapping catheter often extends into the vein distal to electrically active tissue. The third-generation cryoballoon improves on the second-generation device by having a 40% shorter distal tip (8 mm vs 13 mm), which increased the possibility of recording pulmonary vein electrograms during cryoablation by 29%.[10]

Efficacy and Safety

The efficacy of the first-generation cryoballoon to achieve acute isolation of all 4 pulmonary veins was found to be 83% using the balloon alone, and 97.6% with the additional use of focal cryoablation in the seminal STOP AF (Sustained Treatment Of Paroxysmal Atrial Fibrillation) trial, and long-term efficacy ranged from 59% to 89%.[11,12] The second-generation cryoballoon catheter is observed to have greater efficacy compared to the first-generation system as uniform distribution of cooling mitigates the effect of malalignment of the balloon to the pulmonary vein antra. Achievement of acute PVI as well as long-term freedom from arrhythmia with the second-generation cryoballoon has been reported to be similar to RF catheter ablation for paroxysmal and persistent atrial fibrillation. With regards to safety, cryoballoon is associated with a significantly higher rate of phrenic nerve injury compared with RF ablation across multiple studies.[13-16] The prospective multicenter randomized FIRE AND ICE clinical trial compared the cryoballoon catheter ablation with RF catheter ablation to treat paroxysmal atrial fibrillation. Kuck and colleagues[17] found no significant difference between the 2 approaches with regards to both safety and efficacy. Acute PVI rates were similar between the RF and cryoballoon arms (97.9% vs 98.9%) and 12-month follow-up with regards to the combined end point of freedom from recurrent atrial arrhythmia, antiarrhythmic medication, or repeat ablation (64.1% vs 65.4%). The investigators found that procedure time (140.9 ± 54.9 vs 124.4 ± 39.0) and left atrial dwell time (108.6 ± 44.9 vs 92.3 ± 31.4) were significantly less in the cryoballoon arm, but total fluoroscopy time was higher (16.6 ± 17.8 vs 21.7 ± 13.9). The cryoballoon arm had a statistically significantly higher rate of phrenic nerve injury at discharge (2.7 vs 0%), although at 12 months this difference was not significant. Although a significant number of patients had ablation performed using a first-generation cryoballoon catheter and non–force-sensing RF ablation catheter, there was no significant difference between the catheters.

Many of the risks of cryoballoon ablation for atrial fibrillation overlap with risks associated with RF catheter ablation, including cardiac, vascular, neurologic, and gastrointestinal complications. Because of the thermal nature of cryoablation, damage to surrounding structures is important, particularly the esophagus and phrenic nerve. Phrenic nerve injury has been observed to be more common with cryoballoon ablation compared with RF point-by-point ablation. Phrenic nerve injury can occur when ablation is performed to isolate the right pulmonary veins because of the proximity of the right phrenic nerve to the superior vena cava (SVC) and the anterior inferior aspect of the right superior pulmonary vein (RSPV), although left phrenic nerve injury during cryoablation of the left pulmonary veins has also been described.[18,19] Techniques to mitigate the risk should be used routinely to avoid permanent phrenic nerve palsy. The most common strategy to assess phrenic nerve injury on the right side is palpating to assess diaphragmatic excursion while pacing the phrenic nerve. The right phrenic nerve is paced from the SVC at twice the capture threshold during ablation of the right pulmonary veins. In addition, the compound motor action potential can be recorded and monitored by placing a quadripolar electrophysiology catheter in the subdiaphragmatic vein to assess for phrenic injury that may improve safety beyond palpation alone.[20,21] Injury to the esophagus with cryoballoon is rare and has been observed to be associated with ablation in the left inferior pulmonary vein and with longer ablation duration. John and colleagues[22] found 11 cases from a pool of 120,000 cases from the Manufacturer and User Facility Device Experience database, publications, and the manufacturer's database, representing less than 0.1% of cases. Balloon inflation times were significantly longer in patients with fistula (238.8 $\pm$ 54.8 seconds vs 178.1 $\pm$ 37.5 seconds in the non-atrioesophageal fistula group, $P \leq .001$). Although not demonstrated in this study, the risk of injury is also thought to increase when balloon nadir temperature exceeds $-60°C$, so should be avoided. Endoluminal esophageal temperature monitoring during ablation may also be of benefit to alert operators of potential thermal risk to the esophagus.

Improving Outcomes

The optimal technique to create durable lesions with cryoballoon has been evaluated in several studies. Several parameters have been identified to be important, including occlusion of the vein, rate of freeze, nadir temperature, time to effect, and thaw time. In a study of 66 patients with the first-generation cryoballoon, Fürnkranz and colleagues[23] reported that a minimal cryoballoon temperature of less than $-51°C$ was associated with successful PVI with 97% specificity, whereas a temperature greater than or equal to $-36°C$ superior/$-33°C$ inferior predicted failed PVI with 95% specificity. The authors' practice has aimed for a target temperature of $-40°C$ to ensure efficacy. Aryana and colleagues[9] analyzed data from 435 PVs in 112 patients who underwent repeat ablation procedures after an index cryoballoon PVI with 111 veins (25.5%) reconnected at follow-up. The important differences between isolated and reconnected veins included time to effect ≤ 60 seconds and interval thaw time of ≥ 10 seconds and were significant predictors of durable PVI. TTI with the second-generation balloon can be determined in 71% to 79% of targeted veins in clinical trials. The utility of this parameter as an independent predictor of recurrent arrhythmia has been validated in several other studies.[24,25]

In addition to improving efficacy, a TTI-guided approach may reduce collateral injury to surrounding structures. In the MADE-PVI study, Cordes and colleagues[26] performed esophagogastroduodenoscopy and endoscopic ultrasound in 70 patients who underwent ablation with a TTI-guided approach or a conventional strategy. They found that there was more edema present in patients undergoing conventional approach (17 mm vs 11 mm, 26% vs 6%) and a higher incidence of esophageal lesions (9% vs 0%). The TTI cohort required significantly less ablation time (211 $\pm$ 84 seconds vs 360 $\pm$ 42 seconds). Of note, in patients who were unable to have TTI assessed, a single 180-second lesion was performed; the investigators did not report how many patients were unable to have TTI demonstrated.

ICE is widely used for complex electrophysiology procedures. The use of ICE to guide cryoballoon ablation was evaluated in a pilot study of 43 patients randomized to ICE and fluoroscopy or fluoroscopy alone. The investigators were able to visualize 80% of ICE-guided freezes with excellent quality. They found that an ICE-guided approach resulted in shorter procedure times (130 $\pm$ 19 minutes vs 143 $\pm$ 27 minutes, $P = .05$) and fluoroscopy times (26 $\pm$ 10 minutes vs 42 $\pm$ 13 minutes, $P = .01$). The investigators also found that the amount of contrast used in the procedure was significantly lower in patients with ICE guidance (88 ± 31 mL vs 169 ± 38 mL).[27] Ottaviano and colleagues[28] performed a feasibility study using real-time 3-dimensional transesophageal echocardiography (TEE) to guide cryoballoon ablation in 45 patients. They were able to use TEE for all 190 targeted veins, which aided them in identifying leaks. They achieved isolation in all targeted veins with a median procedure time of 145 minutes and fluoroscopy time of 24 minutes.

Cryoballoon for Ablation of Extrapulmonary Vein Targets

Recently, there is increased interest in empiric left atrial posterior wall isolation (PWI) in addition to PVI for persistent atrial fibrillation, although the benefit has not been conclusively demonstrated.[29–31] Aryana and colleagues[32] examined the efficacy and safety of PVI and PWI compared with PVI alone using cryoballoon ablation in 390 patients. The investigators achieved PVI and PWI in 99.8% of patients; PWI required 13.7 ± 3.2 applications (34 ± 10 minutes) of cryoablation, and adjunctive RF ablation was required in 32.4% of cases. The investigators observed that PVI and PWI were associated with greater atrial fibrillation termination (19.8% vs 8.9%, $P = .003$) and conversion to atrial flutter (12.2% vs 5.4%, $P = .02$). At 12 months follow-up, recurrence of atrial fibrillation and all atrial arrhythmias was lower in the combined PVI and PWI group compared with PVI alone (80.2% vs 51.2%, hazard ratio: 2.04, $P = .015$). The investigators conclude that PWI to PVI is feasible with cryoballoon, although RF ablation may be necessary as was the case in a third of patients in their series.

A novel cryoballoon catheter (Cryterion, Boston Scientific, Marlborough, MA, USA) under development is undergoing clinical trials. It is characterized by ability to achieve ultralow temperature and a more compliant material.

- The cryoballoon is a well-validated alternative to RF catheter ablation to achieve PVI. The second-generation device has been demonstrated to achieve a high rate of acute PVI, and long-term follow-up shows similar efficacy to RF ablation.
- A TTI-guided approach may improve efficacy in terms of durable PVI.
- Cryoballoon ablation procedures compared with standard RF ablation for PVI may be shorter with less left atrial dwell time, but require longer fluoroscopy time.
- Safety of cryoballoon is similar to RF ablation, but the rate of phrenic nerve injury in particular

is significantly higher so additional monitoring and continuous assessment during ablation are required.
- Left atrial PWI is feasible with cryoballoon, but additional RF ablation is often required.

LASER BALLOON

The visually guided laser balloon (VGLB; HeartLight; CardioFocus Inc, Marlborough, MA, USA) is a clinically available ablation catheter that includes a 2F endoscope to allow direct visualization of pulmonary vein and creates thermal lesions using a 980-nm laser light (**Fig. 1**).

Technology and Technique

The first-generation device comprises a noncompliant balloon available in 3 sizes (20, 25, and 30 mm) and delivered energy in large 90° to 150° arcs. The second-generation catheter was modified to include a compliant, variable diameter balloon and deliver energy in 30° maneuverable arcs. The balloon, which is filled with deuterium oxide (D_2O), is compliant and modifiable to 7 sizes to allow greater contact and occlusion of a variety of pulmonary vein ostia. Conceptually, direct visualization of the pulmonary veins enables operators to (1) avoid ablating within veins, which would increase risk of pulmonary vein stenosis and leaving proximal triggers of atrial fibrillation unaffected; and (2) ensure complete vein occlusion so laser energy is not applied to blood, which could result in thrombus formation.[33,34] Direct lesion visualization via the endoscope is feasible, but in animal models was demonstrated to be unreliable, and electroanatomical mapping with a multipolar catheter to assess for PVI after ablation is recommended.

The VGLB catheter is placed in the left atrium through a 12F deflectable sheath. Similar to the cryoballoon, the balloon must be prepared in a saline bath to ensure no air is introduced to the left atrium. After inflation, the device is positioned at the ostium of the target pulmonary vein under fluoroscopic guidance. The catheter has a "Z"-shaped radiopaque orientation marker at the proximal neck of the balloon, which provides rotational orientation of the balloon with respect to endoscopic views so the operator is aware of the visual "blind spot." The blind spot from the endoscopic view is due to the central lumen and is opposite to the orientation marker. In an anteroposterior fluoroscopic view, a "Z" is visualized when the catheter is oriented anterior, and a reverse "Z" is visualized when it is posterior. A half-box on the superior aspect of the catheter indicates a

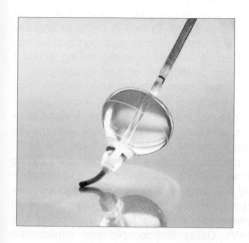

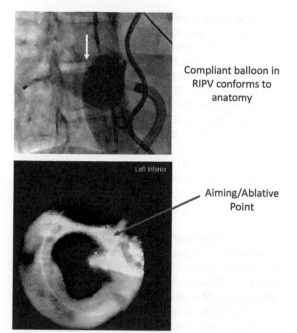

Compliant balloon in RIPV conforms to anatomy

Aiming/Ablative Point

Left Inferior

Fig. 1. The VGLB (HeartLight; CardioFocus Inc) is a clinically available ablation catheter that includes a 2F endo-scope to allow direct visualization of pulmonary vein and creates thermal lesions using a 980 nm laser light. The arrow points to where ablation is being performed, as indicated by the green crescent-shaped light. RIPV, right inferior pulmonary vein. (*Courtesy of* CardioFocus Inc., Marlborough, MA; with permission.)

superior position, and a half-box on the inferior aspect of the catheter indicates an inferior posi-tion. Once adequately positioned, ablation is per-formed circumferentially around the pulmonary vein ostia with overlapping lesions. Laser light at 980-nm wavelength is not absorbed by D_2O and results in volumetric heating of tissue.[35] The dose of laser energy is titratable. In clinical studies, the dose ranged from 5.5 W to 12 W for 20- to 30-second duration. Varying the power was deter-mined by the operator based on factors such as presence of blood in the endoscopic field of view and thickness of tissue (ie, anterior vs posterior wall).

Efficacy and Safety

The second-generation laser balloon has been found to have similar efficacy outcomes for acute PVI compared with RF ablation. In terms of safety, studies have shown phrenic nerve injury to be significantly higher with laser balloon. Effi-cacy as well as procedure length and fluoroscopy use is linked to operator experience. The Heart-Light Study was the first major randomized multi-center trial comparing safety and efficacy of the second-generation VGLB to RF ablation. Three hundred fifty-three patients with symptomatic

paroxysmal atrial fibrillation were randomized to either VGLB or standard RF ablation with a non–force-sensing irrigated ablation catheter and fol-lowed for 12 months. The investigators achieved acute isolation in 99.7% of targeted PVs in the VGLB group compared with 99.1% in the RF ablation group (*P* = .05). At 12 months, the pri-mary efficacy outcome of freedom from docu-mented atrial fibrillation, atrial flutter, failure to acutely isolate all PV, repeat ablation, or use of antiarrhythmic therapy was similar in the VGLB and RF ablation group (61.1% vs 61.7%, *P* = .003 for noninferiority). In terms of safety out-comes, the laser balloon arm was observed to have significantly higher rate of diaphragmatic paralysis (3.5% vs 0.6%, *P* = .05) despite a pro-tocol of phrenic pacing during ablation of the RSPV. The fluoroscopy (35.6 ± 18.2 vs 29.7 ± 21.0), ablation (173.8 ± 46.6 vs 151.2 ± 56.2), and overall procedure times (236.0 ± 52.8 vs 193.0 ± 63.6) were longer in the VGLB arm compared with the control arm. Of note, the overall procedure time and fluoros-copy time were significantly lower in operators with greater experience (≥15 cases vs <15 cases) in an analysis of operator experience.[36] Several nonrandomized studies have been published demonstrating similarly high rates of acute PVI achieved with the VGLB and improvement in procedure duration with experience.[37-39] In a metaanalysis of 17 studies including 1188 patients, Reynolds and colleagues[40] found that acute PVI was achieved in 98.8% of targeted veins. The pooled estimate for 12-month freedom from atrial arrhythmia in patients with paroxysmal atrial fibrillation was 74.3%. The learning curve effects on procedure duration was analyzed from 5 studies and demonstrated a greater than 60-minute decline in procedure time comparing earliest to most recent procedures. The investigators also reported the rate of phrenic nerve injury was 2.6%.[41]

The third-generation VGLB (X3) has several technological advantages over the second-generation device. The balloon design has been further modified to be continuously and dynamically adjustable to improve contact and ensure level of isolation is optimized. Most notable, an integrated motor has been added to automate circumferential lesion creation, which is anticipated to increase speed and efficacy. The X3 clinical trial results are forthcoming, but preliminary results suggest shorter procedure time with less fluoroscopy.

- The VGLB is an effective alternative to standard RF ablation to achieve PVI with similar safety outcomes, although risk of phrenic injury is higher.
- Direct visualization of pulmonary vein ostia during ablation may reduce risk of pulmonary vein stenosis.
- Compared with cryoballoon, the variable size and compliance may allow for the VGLB to conform to a wider array of pulmonary vein morphologies. Although not compared directly, procedural and fluoroscopy time using cryoballoon is less than laser balloon.

OTHER BALLOON CATHETER SYSTEMS
Hot Balloon

The RF hot balloon (Toray-Satake balloon; Toray Industries, Inc, Tokyo, Japan) is composes of a 12F shaft containing a 3F inner tube and a semicompliant balloon tip available in 1.5-, 2.0-, 2.5-, and 3.0-diameter sizes. An electrode within the balloon delivers unipolar RF energy at a very high frequency (13.56 MHz) to heat fluid within the balloon (a 1:1 mix of saline and contrast) up to 80°C and cause capacitive thermal injury to tissue. The hot balloon is advanced over a wire and adequate contact with the ostial tissue can be assessed by injecting contrast through the catheter lumen to ensure vein occlusion.[42] The second-generation catheter has been updated to include a more compliant balloon that can be inflated up to 25 to 35 mm in order to improve contact with tissue, and an agitation system has been updated so fluid is mixed during ablation and uniform application of heat is achieved. In addition, the second-generation balloon has reduced frequency of RF energy from 13.56 to 1.8 MHz to reduce current leakage. Balloon temperature is maintained 40°C to 70°C with the aid of a thermocouple inside the balloon. The catheter is manipulated via a 13F deflectable guiding sheath to facilitate ablation of PVs and extrapulmonary vein targets.[43] Sohara and colleagues[43] reported outcomes in 100 patients with paroxysmal and persistent atrial fibrillation undergoing PVI and PWI. Using fluoroscopic and intracardiac echocardiographic guidance, the balloon catheter was initially dragged across the left atrial posterior roof, followed by antral ablation of pulmonary vein with wedge occlusion, and then followed by dragging the balloon across the posterior wall between the inferior veins. The energy and ablation duration varied by location, ranging from 5.7 ± 2.1 minutes (Right inferior pulmonary vein (RIPV)) to 10 ± 2.7 minutes (left superior pulmonary vein (LSPV)). Acute isolation of all pulmonary veins and the posterior wall was achieved in all patients. At 11 ± 4.8 months follow-up, 92 out of 100 patients remained free of atrial fibrillation without antiarrhythmic drugs. There were no long-term complications reported, other than 3 asymptomatic pulmonary vein stenoses less than 50%.

High-Intensity Focused Ultrasound

The high-intensity focused ultrasound balloon catheter (HIFU; ProRhythm, Ronkonkoma, NY, USA) is a steerable system comprising a distal noncompliant fluid-filled balloon (water and contrast in a 6:1 ratio) and an integrated 9-MHz ultrasound crystal, and a proximal second noncompliant balloon filled with carbon dioxide. The catheter is designed to deliver nontitratable ultrasound energy in a focused ring ~4 mm distal to the balloon's surface. The catheter is available in 24-, 27-, and 32-mm-diameter sizes. It is inserted over a wire into the target pulmonary vein, and contrast may be injected through a central lumen for pulmonary vein angiography to ensure contact. In an initial study of 15 patients, Schmidt and colleagues[44] achieved acute PVI in 41 of 46 (89%) targeted veins. Two patients had right-sided phrenic nerve palsy despite pacing that did not resolve after 12 months. In a follow-up study of 32 patients with paroxysmal atrial fibrillation that underwent HIFU ablation, 87% of targeted PVs were acutely isolated. At a median follow-up of 1400 days, 56% of patients remained free of atrial fibrillation without antiarrhythmic therapy.[45] The HIFU ablation was discontinued because of reports of 4 severe esophageal complications, which included an atrioesophageal fistula.[46]

Radiofrequency Balloon Catheters

Several multielectrode RF balloon catheters are undergoing clinical evaluation. These catheters include the Heliostar balloon (Biosense Webster, Irvine, CA, USA), the Luminize balloon (Boston Scientific, Marlborough, MA, USA), and the Kardium Globe (Kardium, Burnaby, BC, Canada).

The Heliostar system is composed of a compliant irrigated balloon catheter with 10 flexible gold surface electrodes capable of delivering RF energy and is used with a generator capable of customizing delivery of energy to each individual electrode in terms of power and duration. The catheter is advanced under fluoroscopic guidance over a wire or a 3F mapping catheter and may also be visualized with the CARTO3 (Biosense Webster) electroanatomical mapping system (**Fig. 2**). Antral contact with pulmonary vein ostia is assessed using pulmonary vein angiography by injecting contrast through a central lumen in the catheter. The results of the

RADIANCE (Pulmonary Vein Isolation with a Novel Multi-electrode Radiofrequency Balloon Catheter that Allows Directionally-Tailored Energy Delivery) first-in-man clinical trial were presented at the Heart Rhythm Society meeting in 2017. The study included 30 patients with paroxysmal atrial fibrillation undergoing ablation with the Helios catheter and showed 100% acute PVI, with reconnection in 2.6% of patients with adenosine/isoproterenol challenge. Mean procedure time was 96.6 minutes, and fluoroscopy time was 4.7 minutes.[47] The STELLAR (Safety and Effectiveness Evaluation of the Multi-Electrode Radiofrequency Balloon Catheter for the Treatment of Symptomatic Paroxysmal Atrial Fibrillation) Investigational Device Exemption (IDE) study is underway currently to further evaluate the use of the Heliostar catheter.

The Luminize balloon system, formerly known as the Apama RF balloon, is an over-the-wire 12.5F irrigated RF balloon catheter with 12 proximal and 6 distal electrodes (**Fig. 3**). The catheter also has 4 cameras and LED illumination to allow direct visualization of pulmonary veins to ensure adequate tissue contact. The AF-FICIENT first-in-human clinical trial of 18 patients was presented at the European Heart Rhythm Association meeting in 2019 and demonstrated successful isolation of 98% of pulmonary veins, and 80% freedom from atrial fibrillation at 6 months.[48]

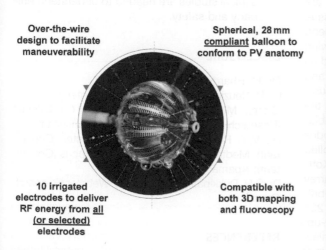

Over-the-wire design to facilitate maneuverability

Spherical, 28 mm <u>compliant</u> balloon to conform to PV anatomy

10 irrigated electrodes to deliver RF energy from <u>all</u> <u>(or selected)</u> electrodes

Compatible with both 3D mapping and fluoroscopy

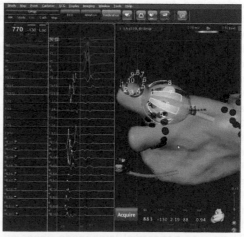

Fig. 2. The Heliostar system is composed of a compliant irrigated balloon catheter with 10 flexible gold surface electrodes capable of delivering RF energy and is used with a generator capable of customizing delivery of energy to each individual electrode in terms of power and duration. The catheter is advanced under fluoroscopic guidance over a wire or a 3F mapping catheter and may also be visualized with the CARTO3 electroanatomical mapping system. 3D, 3-dimensional; PV, pulmonary vein. (*Image provided courtesy* of Boston Scientific. ©2020 Boston Scientific Corporation or its affiliates. All rights reserved.)

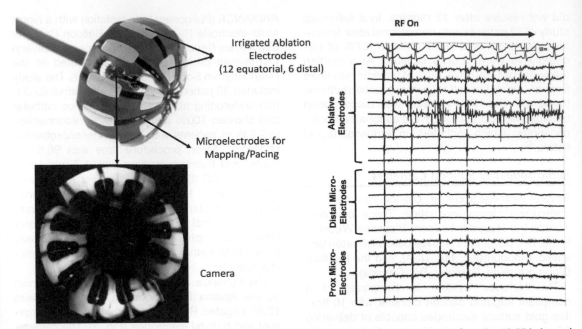

Fig. 3. The Luminize balloon system, formerly known as the Apama RF balloon, is an over-the-wire 12.5F irrigated RF balloon catheter with 12 proximal and 6 distal electrodes. prox, proximal. (*Courtesy of* Boston Scientific, Inc., Marlborough, MA; with permission.)

The Kardium Globe catheter consists of a nonirrigated multielectrode array of 122 gold-plated electrodes ranging from 9.0 to 13.5 mm^2 in size on 16 ribs. Electrodes are each capable of delivering RF energy, pacing, recording electrograms, and measuring current. A temperature sensor 0.025 mm behind the electrode allows for temperature feedback. The individual electrodes are determined to be in contact with atrial tissue based on continuous temperature measurement, whereby the rate of convective cooling by flowing blood creates variation. An "FLOW" map based on contact is used to resolve anatomic features and determine real-time contact, and a continuously updating "WAVE" map shows propagation in the atrium. The system allows for simultaneous ablation with up to 24 individually controlled electrodes simultaneously in a temperature-controlled mode.[49] In the Global Atrial Fibrillation study, Kottkamp and colleagues[50] evaluated the Globe array system in 60 patients with paroxysmal atrial fibrillation. Acute PVI was achieved in 232 of 234 (99.1%) targeted veins. At 12-months' follow-up, there was 72.3% freedom from atrial arrhythmias. There was pericardial tamponade observed in 2 patients related to transseptal puncture and array insertion, but no other serious adverse events reported.

- Balloon-based catheter ablation systems using different energy sources have been developed, but are not widely available. The HIFU balloon device was discontinued because of high risk of complications.
- RF catheter balloons are under development and appear to show great promise, but further clinical studies are needed to understand efficacy and safety.

DISCLOSURE

Dr. R. Bhardwaj, MD: None.
Dr. P. Neuzil, MD, PhD: Biosense-Webster (Research Grant); Medtronic (Research Grant); Cardiofocus (Research Grant); Boston Scientific (Consultant).
Dr. V.Y. Reddy, MD: Biosense-Webster (Consultant); Medtronic (Consultant); Cardiofocus (Consultant); Apama (Consultant, Equity).
Dr. S.R. Dukkipati, MD: Biosense-Webster (Research Grant).

REFERENCES

1. Haïssaguerre M, Jaïs P, Shah DC, et al. Spontaneous initiation of atrial fibrillation by ectopic beats originating in the pulmonary veins. N Engl J Med 1998;339:659–66.

2. Ouyang F, Bänsch D, Ernst S, et al. Complete isolation of left atrium surrounding the pulmonary veins: new insights from the double-Lasso technique in paroxysmal atrial fibrillation. Circulation 2004;110: 2090–6.

3. Reddy VY, Dukkipati SR, Neuzil P, et al. Randomized, controlled trial of the safety and effectiveness of a contact force-sensing irrigated catheter for ablation of paroxysmal atrial fibrillation: results of the TactiCath Contact Force Ablation Catheter Study for Atrial Fibrillation (TOCCASTAR) study. Circulation 2015;132:907–15.

4. Natale A, Reddy VY, Monir G, et al. Paroxysmal AF catheter ablation with a contact force sensing catheter: results of the prospective, multicenter SMART-AF trial. J Am Coll Cardiol 2014;64: 647–56.

5. Kuck KH, Hoffmann BA, Ernst S, et al. Impact of complete versus incomplete circumferential lines around the pulmonary veins during catheter ablation of paroxysmal atrial fibrillation: results from the Gap-Atrial Fibrillation-German Atrial Fibrillation Competence Network 1 Trial. Circ Arrhythm Electrophysiol 2016;9:e003337.

6. Khairy P, Dubuc M. Transcatheter cryoablation part I: preclinical experience. Pacing Clin Electrophysiol 2008;31:112–20.

7. Straube F, Drowarth U, Schmidt M, et al. Comparison of the first and second cryoballoon: high-volume single-center safety and efficacy analysis. Circ Arrhythm Electrophysiol 2014;7:293–9.

8. Di Giovanni G, Wauters K, Chierchia GB, et al. One-year follow-up after single procedure cryoballoon ablation: a comparison between the first and second generation balloon. J Cardiovasc Electrophysiol 2014;25:834–9.

9. Aryana A, Mugnai G, Singh S, et al. Procedural and biophysical indicators of durable pulmonary vein isolation during cryoballoon ablation of atrial fibrillation. Heart Rhythm 2016;13:424–32.

10. Aryana A, Kowalski M, O'Neill PG, et al. Catheter ablation using the third-generation cryoballoon provides an enhanced ability to assess time to pulmonary vein isolation facilitating the ablation strategy: short- and long-term results of a multicenter study. Heart Rhythm 2016;13:2306–13.

11. Packer DL, Kowal RC, Wheelan KR, et al. Cryoballoon ablation of pulmonary veins for paroxysmal atrial fibrillation: first results of the North American Arctic Front (STOP AF) pivotal trial. J Am Coll Cardiol 2013;61:1713–23.

12. Aryana A, Morkoch S, Bailey S, et al. Acute procedural and cryoballoon characteristics from cryoablation of atrial fibrillation using the first- and second-generation cryoballoon: a retrospective comparative study with follow-up outcomes. J Interv Card Electrophysiol 2014;41:177–86.

13. Pandya B, Sheikh A, Spagnola J, et al. Safety and efficacy of second-generation versus first-generation cryoballoons for treatment of atrial fibrillation: a meta-analysis of current evidence. J Interv Card Electrophysiol 2016;45:49–56.

14. Su W, Orme GJ, Hoyt R, et al. Retrospective review of arctic front advance cryoballoon ablation: a multicenter examination of second-generation cryoballoon (RADICOOL trial). J Interv Card Electrophysiol 2018;51:199–204.

15. Buiatti A, von Olshausen G, Barthel P, et al. Cryoballoon vs. radiofrequency ablation for paroxysmal atrial fibrillation: an updated meta-analysis of randomized and observational studies. Europace 2017;19:378–84.

16. Omran H, Gutleben KJ, Molatta S, et al. Second generation cryoballoon ablation for persistent atrial fibrillation: an updated meta-analysis. Clin Res Cardiol 2018;107:182–92.

17. Kuck KH, Brugada J, Fürnkranz A, et al, FIRE AND ICE Investigators. Cryoballoon or radiofrequency ablation for paroxysmal atrial fibrillation. N Engl J Med 2016;374:2235–45.

18. Fürnkranz A, Bordignon S, Schmidt B, et al. Incidence and characteristics of phrenic nerve palsy following pulmonary vein isolation with the second-generation as compared with the first-generation cryoballoon in 360 consecutive patients. Europace 2015;17:574–8.

19. Okishige K, Aoyagi H, Nishimura T, et al. Left phrenic nerve injury during electrical isolation of left-sided pulmonary veins with the second-generation cryoballoon. Pacing Clin Electrophysiol 2017; 40:1426–31.

20. Franceschi F, Dubuc M, Guerra PG, et al. Phrenic nerve monitoring with diaphragmatic electromyography during cryoballoon ablation for atrial fibrillation: the first human application. Heart Rhythm 2011;8:1068–71.

21. Franceschi F, Koutbi L, Mancini J, et al. Novel electromyographic monitoring technique for prevention of right phrenic nerve palsy during cryoballoon ablation. Circ Arrhythm Electrophysiol 2013;6: 1109–14.

22. John RM, Kapur S, Ellenbogan KA, et al. Atrioesophageal fistula formation with cryoballoon ablation is commonly related to the left inferior pulmonary vein. Heart Rhythm 2017;14:184–9.

23. Fürnkranz A, Köster I, Julian Chun KR, et al. Cryoballoon temperature predicts acute pulmonary vein isolation. Heart Rhythm 2011;8:821–5.

24. Reissmann B, Wissner E, Deiss S, et al. First insights into cryoballoon-based pulmonary vein isolation taking the individual time-to-isolation into account. Europace 2017;19:1676–80.

25. Julian Chun KR, Stich M, Fürnkranz A, et al. Individualized cryoballoon energy pulmonary vein isolation guided by real-time pulmonary vein recordings, the randomized ICE-T trial. Heart Rhythm 2017;14: 495–500.

26. Cordes F, Ellermann C, Dechering DG, et al. Time-to-isolation-guided cryoballoon ablation reduces oesophageal and mediastinal alterations detected by endoscopic ultrasound: results of the MADE-PVI trial. Europace 2019;21:1325–33.

27. Schmidt M, Daccarett M, Marschang H, et al. Intracardiac echocardiography improves procedural efficiency during cryoballoon ablation for atrial fibrillation: a pilot study. J Interv Card Electrophysiol 2010;21:1202–7.

28. Ottaviano L, Chierchia GB, Bregasi A, et al. Cryoballoon ablation for atrial fibrillation guided by real-time three-dimensional transoesophageal echocardiography: a feasibility study. Europace 2013;15:944–50.

29. Bai R, Di Biase L, Mohanty P, et al. Proven isolation of the pulmonary vein antrum with or without left atrial posterior wall isolation in patients with persistent atrial fibrillation. Heart Rhythm 2016;13:132–40.

30. Verma A, Jiang C, Betts TR, et al. Approaches to catheter ablation for persistent atrial fibrillation. N Engl J Med 2015;372:1812–22.

31. Thiyagaraja A, Kadhim K, Lau DH, et al. Feasibility, safety, and efficacy of posterior wall isolation during atrial fibrillation ablation: a systematic review and meta-analysis. Circ Arrhythm Electrophysiol 2019; 12:e007005.

32. Aryana A, Baker JH, Espinosa Ginic MA, et al. Posterior wall isolation using the cryoballoon in conjunction with pulmonary vein ablation is superior to pulmonary vein isolation alone in patients with persistent atrial fibrillation: a multicenter experience. Heart Rhythm 2018;15:1121–9.

33. Reddy VY, Neuzil P, Themistoclakis S, et al. Visually-guided balloon catheter ablation of atrial fibrillation: experimental feasibility and first-in-human multicenter clinical outcome. Circulation 2009;120: 12–20.

34. Dukkipati SR, Neuzil P, Skoda J, et al. Visual balloon-guided point-by-point ablation: reliable, reproducible, and persistent pulmonary vein isolation. Circ Arrhythm Electrophysiol 2010;3:266–73.

35. Reddy VY, Houghtaling C, Fallon J, et al. Use of a diode laser balloon ablation catheter to generate circumferential pulmonary venous lesions in an open-thoracotomy caprine model. Pacing Clin Electrophysiol 2004;27:52–7.

36. Dukkipati SR, Cuoco F, Kutinsky I, et al, for the HeartLight Study Investigators. Pulmonary vein isolation using the visually guided laser balloon: a prospective, multicenter, and randomized comparison to standard radiofrequency ablation. J Am Coll Cardiol 2015;66:1350–60.

37. Perrotta L, Bordignon S, Dugo D, et al. How to learn pulmonary vein isolation with a novel ablation device: learning curve effects using the endoscopic ablation system. J Cardiovasc Electrophysiol 2014; 25:1293–8.

38. Sediva L, Petru J, Skoda J, et al. Visually guided laser ablation: a single-centre long-term experience. Europace 2014;16:1746–51.

39. Dukkipati SR, Kuck KH, Neuzi P, et al. Pulmonary vein isolation using a visually guided laser balloon catheter: the first 200-patient multicenter clinical experience. Circ Arrhythm Electrophysiol 2013;6: 467–72.

40. Reynolds MR, Zheng Q, Doros G. Laser balloon ablation for AF: a systematic review and meta-analysis. J Cardiovasc Electrophysiol 2018;29:1363–70.

41. Nagase T, Bordignon S, Perrotta L, et al. HEartLight guided–PUre pulmonary vein isolation regardless of concomitant atrial substrate: HEURECA study. Pacing Clin Electrophysiol 2019;42:22–30.

42. Tanaka K, Satake S, Saito S, et al. A new radiofrequency thermal balloon catheter for pulmonary vein isolation. J Am Coll Cardiol 2001;38:2079–86.

43. Sohara H, Takeda H, Ueno H, et al. Feasibility of the radiofrequency hot balloon catheter for isolation of the posterior left atrium and pulmonary veins for the treatment of atrial fibrillation. Circ Arrhythm Electrophysiol 2009;2:225–32.

44. Schmidt B, Antz M, Ernst S, et al. Pulmonary vein isolation by high-intensity focused ultrasound: first-in-man study with a steerable balloon catheter. Heart Rhythm 2007;4:575–84.

45. Metzner A, Julian Chun KR, Neven K, et al. Long-term clinical outcome following pulmonary vein isolation with high-intensity focused ultrasound balloon catheters in patients with paroxysmal atrial fibrillation. Europace 2010;12:188–93.

46. Borchert B, Lawrenz T, Hansky B, et al. Lethal atrioesophageal fistula after pulmonary vein isolation using high-intensity focused ultrasound (HIFU). Heart Rhythm 2008;5:145–8.

47. Reddy VY, Schilling RJ, Grimaldi, et al. PV isolation with a novel multielectrode radiofrequency balloon catheter that allows directionally tailored energy delivery (RADIANCE): a multicenter first-in-man experience. Heart Rhythm 2017;14:948–50 (C-LBCT03-04).

48. Al-Ahmad A, Natale A, Reddy VY, et al. Real-time contact visualization via built-in cameras improves

lesion quality in multi-electrode radiofrequency (RF) balloon catheter ablation during pulmonary vein isolation in humans. Heart Rhythm 2017;14(No. 5). PO02-58 S166-16.

49. Kottkamp H, Moser F, Rieger A, et al. Global multi-electrode contact mapping plus ablation with a single catheter: preclinical and preliminary experience in humans with atrial fibrillation. J Cardiovasc Electrophysiol 2017;28:1247-56.

50. Kottkamp H, Hindricks G, Pönisch C, et al. Global multielectrode contact-mapping plus ablation with a single catheter in patients with atrial fibrillation: Global AF study. J Cardiovasc Electrophysiol 2019; 30:2248–55.

Recurrent Atrial Fibrillation After Radiofrequency Ablation
What to Expect

Tharian S. Cherian, MD, David J. Callans, MD*

KEYWORDS

- Atrial fibrillation • Radiofrequency ablation • Recurrence • Pulmonary vein isolation

KEY POINTS

- Recurrent AF after RF ablation is common, with up to 50% of patients experiencing recurrence within 3 months.
- Early and multiple recurrences are harbingers of late recurrence within 1 year, which occurs in 20% to 50% of the patients, with persistent AF patients experiencing worse outcomes.
- Although no consensus exists regarding patient selection and timing of redo ablation, we refer symptomatic patients with multiple recurrences and persistent AF for redo ablation.
- Reisolation of the frequently encountered reconnected pulmonary veins and ablation of non-PV triggers is our primary ablation strategy for recurrent AF.
- We recommend aggressive lifestyle modifications including weight loss, treatment of sleep-disordered breathing, and management of comorbid conditions for durable maintenance of sinus rhythm.

INTRODUCTION

Radiofrequency (RF) catheter ablation is an effective treatment strategy for atrial fibrillation (AF), and in particular is a guideline recommended therapy for symptomatic AF. Following the seminal work by Haissaguerre and coworkers,[1] who demonstrated pulmonary vein (PV) triggers for AF, PV isolation (PVI) has become the initial strategy for patients with AF referred for catheter ablation. One of the challenging aspects of managing patients postablation is the commonly encountered phenomena of AF recurrence. In this article, we describe the epidemiology of early, late, and long-term recurrences of AF after ablation; outline risk factors and monitoring strategies for recurrence; review management options; highlight the importance of lifestyle modifications; and layout our general approach to redo ablation in patients who experience recurrence.

EARLY RECURRENCE OF ATRIAL FIBRILLATION AFTER RADIOFREQUENCY ABLATION
Epidemiology of Early Recurrence of Atrial Fibrillation and Implications for Late Recurrence

Early recurrence of AF after ablation is commonly encountered in clinical practice. Observational studies have used "blanking periods," which are designated time intervals immediately following ablation, ranging from 48 hours to 3 months to quantify early recurrence. These studies report

Cardiovascular Division, Electrophysiology Section, Hospital of the University of Pennsylvania, 9.129 Founders Pavilion, 3400 Spruce Street, Philadelphia PA 19104, USA
* Corresponding author.
E-mail address: david.callans@uphs.upenn.edu
Twitter: @tscherian (T.S.C.); @DavidCallans (D.J.C.)

Card Electrophysiol Clin 12 (2020) 187–197
https://doi.org/10.1016/j.ccep.2020.02.003
1877-9182/20/© 2020 Elsevier Inc. All rights reserved.

that 25% to 65% of patients undergoing an ablation procedure for AF experience early recurrence.[2] They have also shown that early recurrence is a nonspecific predictor of late recurrence, with approximately half the patients with early recurrence remaining free of AF during long-term follow-up (**Table 1**). Given these findings, the most recent multisociety expert consensus statement recommend a blanking period of 3 months, during which further ablation is not undertaken.[3]

Despite the high incidence of early recurrence in patients with and without late recurrence, early recurrence has been reproducibly associated with late recurrence, and therefore does provide prognostic information regarding long-term ablation success. Lee and colleagues[4] reported in a multivariate analysis that early recurrence could predict late recurrence of AF (hazard ratio, 1.62). In a substudy of the STAR-AF trial, 50% of the patients experienced early and late recurrences defined as recurrence less than 3 months and 3 to 12 months after the procedure, respectively. Early recurrence (hazard ratio, 3.23) was associated with late recurrence.[5]

The timing of early recurrence seems to be an important predictor of late recurrence. Liu and colleagues[6] reported that in patients with successful ablation, early recurrences were infrequent and decreased significantly over time compared with patients who experienced later recurrence. Themistoclakis and colleagues[7] demonstrated that risk of late recurrence was inversely proportional to the timing of first recurrence, with recurrences in the third month being highly predictive of late recurrence. Similarly, Koyama and colleagues[8] found significantly lower 6-month recurrence rate in patients who had experienced early recurrence within 72 hours of the index procedure when compared with those patients who experienced recurrences between 72 hours and a month.

In our experience, the timing and frequency of early recurrence of AF following index ablation does provide valuable information regarding long-term ablation success. Liang and colleagues[9] reported on the predictive value of early recurrence in the first 6 weeks following ablation. In this study, the blanking interval was divided into three 2-week intervals. Early recurrence was associated with worse long-term ablation success (defined as absence of AF >30 seconds off antiarrhythmic drugs [AAD]) at 1 year (40% vs 80%). Multiple recurrences in separate 2-week intervals more strongly predicted long-term ablation failure compared with recurrence in a single 2-week interval.[9]

Atrial Tachycardias and Atrial Flutters After Ablation for Atrial Fibrillation

Although AF is the most frequently observed recurrent arrhythmia, atrial flutters and atrial tachycardias are not uncommon in the postablation period (**Fig. 1**). Areas of conduction block created by left atrial (LA) ablation is well understood to be substrate for these arrhythmias. In the early days of PVI, Gerstenfeld and colleagues[10] reported a 3% incidence of organized LA tachycardia following ablation. Most of these tachycardias were of focal origin in the reconnected segments of PVs and redo catheter ablation was curative in most of these patients. In the modern era, LA macroreentrant tachycardias are most commonly associated with substrate ablation techniques, in particular linear lesions during the index ablation. The incidence of these arrhythmias following catheter ablation is variable in the reported literature, because it depends on the method and extent of ablation, and on the underlying LA substrate. The incidence of LA organized tachycardias ranges from 10% to 40% in complex fractionated electrogram (CFAE) ablation studies and other substrate-based ablation studies.[11–13] In practice, most post-AF ablation flutters are mitral annular flutters and roof flutters from the LA, cavotricuspid isthmus–dependent right atrial flutter, less commonly PV atrial tachycardias, and rarely interatrial septal flutters or other focal or microreentrant tachycardia. In our experience, catheter ablation is potentially curative in most of these patients.

Monitoring Strategies for Early Recurrence

Detecting AF recurrences is critical to management of patients in the postablation period. Most of the studies of AF recurrence used Holter monitors or mobile continuous outpatient telemetry devices prompted by patient symptoms or at prespecified time intervals to detect and quantify recurrence (see **Table 1**). In our practice, most patients are routinely monitored by a 30-day mobile continuous outpatient telemetry device in the first few weeks following ablation, at 6 months, and at 1 year or prompted by symptoms. More recently, implantable loop recorders have been used to document arrhythmia recurrence in a more comprehensive and continuous fashion. Continuous monitoring is particularly crucial in patients who are potentially candidates for discontinuation of anticoagulation therapy should maintenance of sinus rhythm be achieved in the long term. In the observational LINQ AF study designed to study the device detection metrics, 419 patients undergoing catheter ablation for AF

Table 1
Selected studies of early and late recurrences of atrial fibrillation after radiofrequency ablation

Study	N	Parox (%)	Pers (%)	Ablation Strategy	Recurrence Definition	ER Time Frame	ER (%)	LR (%)	% ER with LR	Monitoring
Oral et al,[53] 2002	110	85	15	PVI	ECG documented symptomatic AF	2 wk	35	34	69	Symptom-based event recording
Lee et al,[4] 2004	207	100	0	PVI ± LAFW, CT, LM	ECG documented symptomatic AF	1 mo	39	34	43	Symptom-based
Della Bella et al,[54] 2005	263	78	22	PVI ± CTI	ECG documented AF	72 h	24	—	—	TTM daily × 8 wk, Holter q 3 mo
Bertaglia et al,[55] 2005	143	45	55	PVI ± CTI, MAL	ECG documented AT/AF >30 s	3 mo	46	29	57	Holter q 3 mo
Richter et al,[56] 2008	234	70	30	PVI ± RL, MAL	ECG documented AT/AF >30 s	48 h	43	41	54	48-h monitor, Holter 6 w, q 3 mo
Themistoclakis et al,[7] 2008	1298	54	46	PVI + SVC	ECG documented AT/AF >1 min	3 mo	40	22	52	48-h Holter 1, 3, 6, 9, 12 mo
Joshi et al,[65] 2009	72	67	33	PVI ± RL, MAL	ECG documented AF >30 s	3 mo	65	43	62	Event monitor 3 mo, TTM, loop, ECG
Arya et al,[57] 2010	674	85	15	PVI ± RL, MAL	ECG documented AT/AF >30 s	1 wk	52	26	41	7-d Holter q 3 mo
Choi et al,[58] 2010	352	—	—	PVI ± MAL, RL, CTI	ECG documented AT/AF >30 s	3 mo	16	16	41	Holter 3, 6, 12 mo
Verma et al,[59] 2010	100	64	36	PVI and CFE	ECG documented AF >30 s	3 mo	49	49	67	48-h Holter 3, 6, 12 mo
Liang et al,[9] 2015	300	33	67	PVI + triggers	AF >30 s	6 wk	53	44	80	MCOT for symptoms, 6 mo, 1 y

Abbreviations: AT, atrial tachycardia; CFE, complex fractionated electrogram; CT, crista terminalis; CTI, cavotricuspid isthmus; ECG, electrocardiogram; ER, early recurrence; LAFW, left atrial free wall; LM, ligament of Marshall; LR, late recurrence; MAL, mitral annular line; MCOT, mobile continuous outpatient telemetry; N, number of patients; Parox, paroxysmal; Pers, persistent; RL, roof line; SVC, superior vena cava; TTM, transtelephonic monitoring.
Adapted from Andrade JG, Khairy P, Verma A et al. Early recurrence of atrial tachyarrhythmias following radiofrequency catheter ablation of atrial fibrillation. Pacing Clin Electrophysiol 2012;35:106-16; with permission.

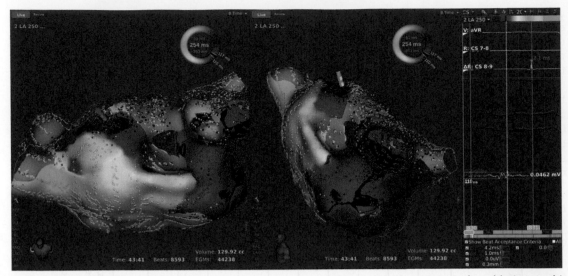

Fig. 1. Left atrial organized tachycardias are not uncommon in patients with recurrent AF after ablation. In this patient with recurrent, persistent AF with a history of mechanical mitral valve and prior ablation, electrophysiology study was notable for a reconnected right superior pulmonary vein, and a figure-of-eight flutter, specifically a roof flutter through a narrow channel. Ablation here terminated the tachycardia, and patient remained free of AF recurrence at long-term follow-up.

were implanted with the LINQ loop recorder device. AF recurrence was analyzed using four methods: (1) continuous recurrence analysis, (2) discontinuous recurrence analysis, (3) AF-burden analysis, and (4) analysis of individual rhythm profiles. This study found that patients with exclusive short AF episodes (<6 minutes) were rare, and the authors suggested an AF detection duration greater than 6 minutes and AF burden greater than 0.1% as clinically relevant recurrence in patients undergoing loop recorder implantation for postablation monitoring.[14]

Prevention Strategies for Early Atrial Fibrillation Recurrence

Studies have assessed whether AAD in the blanking period may reduce early recurrences, need for hospitalizations and cardioversions, and improve long-term ablation success. The Antiarrhythmic After Ablation of Atrial Fibrillation (5A) Study randomized patients undergoing catheter ablation for paroxysmal AF to AAD versus no AAD 6 weeks after the procedure. There was a significant reduction of early recurrence in the AAD group (19% vs 42%), in the first 6 weeks.[15] In a follow-up of the 5A Study at 6 months, short-term AAD did not improve freedom from late recurrence (72% vs 68%).[16] Similarly, the AMIO-CAT trial randomized patients to amiodarone in the postablation period for 8 weeks and reported that although amiodarone use did not reduce primary end point of recurrence (atrial arrhythmia >30 seconds after the first

3 months) at 6 months, it reduced hospitalizations and need for cardioversions in the blanking period.[17] A larger randomized controlled trial (RCT) of more than 2000 patients, the EAST-AF trial, randomized patients to class I or III AADs for 90 days postablation, and similarly reported significant reduction in recurrent AF in the blanking period, and no significant difference in AF recurrence at 1 year.[18] A subsequent meta-analysis of RCTs evaluating the efficacy of AADs in the blanking period did not show a significant reduction in recurrence.[19] Thus, AADs seem to be an appropriate short-term strategy to manage symptomatic recurrences, and is not a durable strategy for maintenance of sinus rhythm, which may require an additional procedure to achieve.

The inflammatory hypothesis regarding the mechanism of early recurrence has led to multiple studies evaluating steroid therapy in the postablative period to reduce recurrence. These studies have yielded mixed results with one randomized study showing reduced recurrence in the first 3 days and at 14 months of follow-up,[20] whereas the other showed reduced early recurrence at 3 months and no difference at 24-month follow-up.[21] A more recent RCT showed no significant improvement in early or late recurrence at 1 year, despite improvement in inflammatory markers.[22]

The effect of the anti-inflammatory medication colchicine on recurrence has been studied in randomized trials in patients undergoing AF ablation. In the first of two trials by Deftereos and colleagues,[23] patients randomized to the colchicine 0.5 mg twice daily group had lower rates of early recurrence during the 3-month follow-up period along with lower inflammatory markers. In the larger follow-up RCT, the colchicine group not only had lower rates of early recurrence, patients also had lower AF recurrence (31% vs 50%; relative risk reduction, 37%; odds ratio, 0.46) over long-term follow-up of 15 months.[24] Larger trials have yet to confirm these results and colchicine use for recurrence prevention has not been adopted into routine practice.

Lifestyle Modifications for Reducing Atrial Fibrillation Recurrence

There is growing evidence that aggressive lifestyle modifications may promote a healthier atrial substrate conducive to maintaining sinus rhythm. The ARREST-AF cohort study offered guideline-recommended risk factor management (weight, blood pressure, blood sugar, lipid, sleep-disordered breathing, smoking, and alcohol) to 69 patients with body mass index greater than or equal to 27 kg/m^2 and at least one cardiac risk factor undergoing AF ablation. When compared with control patients, arrhythmia-free survival after single and multiple procedures was significantly greater in the treatment arm. In addition, risk factor management was an independent predictor of arrhythmia-free survival, associated with five-fold lower risk of AF recurrence over follow-up of 42 months.[25] The authors identified a dose-dependent effect in long-term follow-up in the LEGACY study, with greater than 10% weight loss in a 48-month follow-up period associated with six-fold lower risk of AF recurrence, compared with patients achieving less than 3% weight loss.[26]

In the CARDIO-FIT study, patients with the same profile as the ARREST-AF study were enrolled in a tailored exercise program, and a significant reduction in AF burden and symptom severity were observed in those patients who had a greater than or equal to 2 metabolic equivalents improvement in cardiorespiratory fitness during exercise stress testing compared with those patients without similar improvement. In addition, arrhythmia-free survival was greatest in patients with higher fitness when compared with patients with adequate or low fitness as assessed by exercise stress testing.[27] In a retrospective study, Mohanty and colleagues[28] reported that lifestyle modification, including calorie restriction and moderate physical activity, was associated with similar AF-free survival as a redo catheter ablation procedure in patients experiencing AF recurrence after a first time ablation

procedure. Patient education regarding the importance of lifestyle changes focused on weight loss, exercise, and treatment of sleep-disordered breathing is crucial in preventing and reducing recurrences following ablation.

Repeat Ablation for Early Recurrence

Redo ablation for early recurrence should in theory be informed by the mechanism underlying recurrence. Recurrence in the immediate period following ablation has been postulated to be caused by transient proarrhythmic etiologies, such as inflammatory response of the atrial tissue to RF, changes in the autonomic nervous system, and maturation of the ablative lesions.[3] The self-resolving nature of these etiologies is the rationale behind designation of a blanking period during which pursuing repeat ablation is not recommended. However, should the recurrence be secondary to causes related to AF triggers or substrate (ie, reconnection of the PVs) then a more aggressive ablative approach up front may make more sense. Das and colleagues[29] performed electrophysiology study in 40 patients who underwent PVI for paroxysmal AF, 2 months after the index procedure. Early recurrence of AF in the second month following the procedure was associated with PV reconnection, whereas recurrence in the first month was not. This finding suggests that recurrence in the period immediately following ablation and up to a month may be secondary to transient etiologies, and later recurrences in the currently recommended blanking period may suggest a less durable ablation.

Data regarding optimal timing of redo ablation are sparse. Lellouche and colleagues[30] reported on a subset of patients with early recurrence who underwent redo ablation within the first month of their index procedure. Compared with patients who had redo ablation more than a month from the index procedure, the early reablation group had a lower rate of clinical recurrences, and fewer additional procedures. However, total number of procedures in the long term was greater in the early reablation group.[30] Additional studies are required to define optimal timing for repeat ablation for recurrent AF.

In practice, performing electrophysiology studies to determine the cause of recurrence is not practical. Therefore, it becomes imperative to identify patients with early recurrence who will require a repeat ablation procedure to maintain sinus rhythm in the long term and avoid late recurrences based on clinical characteristics. Our experience is in line with multiple other studies, which have documented that multiple recurrences, particularly occurring later out from the index procedure, and persistent AF in the post-ablation period are predictive of late recurrence. At our center, our practice is to offer such patients (with ongoing indications for ablation therapy) redo ablation even when the recurrences occur within the traditionally defined 3-month blanking period. In addition, patients with atrial flutter or atrial tachycardias who are challenging to rate control in the postablative period are also referred sooner rather than later for electrophysiology study and ablation. We also consider the presence of factors that portend a poor prognosis for sinus rhythm maintenance in making the decision for redo ablation: severely dilated and scarred LA substrate encountered at the index procedure; ongoing risk factors, such as obesity, poorly managed hypertension, and sleep-disordered breathing; and duration of AF.

LATE RECURRENCE OF ATRIAL FIBRILLATION AFTER ABLATION

Late recurrence is defined as AF recurrence between 3 months and 1 year following ablation. Incidence of late recurrence ranges from 20% to 50% (see **Table 1**). Predictors of late recurrence include baseline patient characteristics, such as older age, hypertension, and structural heart disease, and AF characteristics, such as nonparoxysmal AF and longer duration of AF. Characteristics of LA substrate predicting recurrence include dilated LA, presence of diastolic dysfunction, and epicardial LA fat. Procedural findings predicting late recurrence include longer AF ablation time, incomplete PVI, multiple AF foci, and cardioversion required during index ablation procedure (**Table 2**). Late recurrences mechanistically represent ongoing AF triggers that have recurred after initial suppression, inadequately suppressed, or not targeted at the index procedure. As such, our threshold for referring patients with ongoing indications for rhythm control, experiencing late recurrence, to redo ablation is low.

LONG-TERM RECURRENCE OF ATRIAL FIBRILLATION AFTER ABLATION
Epidemiology of Long-Term Recurrence of Atrial Fibrillation After Radiofrequency Ablation

Long-term recurrence is defined as AF recurrence after an AF-free period greater than a year. Similar to studies reporting on early recurrence of AF after RF, there is significant heterogeneity in rates of long-term AF recurrence reported in studies. In addition, many of these studies are older and reflect results before incorporation of modern techniques and technologies. Tzou and colleagues[31] reported our institutional experience on long-term outcome of patients with paroxysmal or persistent AF who had undergone ablation (PVI and non-PV triggers), who were free of AF greater than 1 year following ablation at a single institution. In this cohort, 85% of the patients at 3 years and 71% of patients at 5 years were free of AF, without AAD. Recurrence after 5 years was associated with age, larger LA size, more AF triggers, and persistent AF.[31] Of interest, although the rate of long-term recurrence is discouraging, in many of these patients recurrent episodes were rare and self-limited, often not requiring additional treatment.

In a meta-analysis by Ganesan and colleagues[32] of 19 studies and more than 6000 patients, which included studies that reported on outcomes greater than or equal to 3 years following AF ablation, single procedure success was 54% in paroxysmal AF and 42% in nonparoxysmal AF. With multiple procedures, long-term success approached 80%, and average number of procedures per patient was 1.5.

More recently, Shah and colleagues[33] reported on patients who had recurrence of AF after initial long-term ablation success defined as free from recurrence for greater than 36 months. In this cohort around 1% of the more than 10,000 patients who underwent ablation had a median arrhythmia-free period of 52 months. In patients

Table 2
Predictors of AF recurrence following catheter ablation

Baseline Characteristics	Procedural Characteristics	Imaging and Laboratory Characteristics
Older age[4]	Incomplete PVI[54,55]	Larger LA size[4,7,61,62] (>50 mm[57])
Male gender[57]	Multiple AF foci[4]	LV systolic and diastolic dysfunction[63]
Structural heart disease[4]	AF inducibility[58]	LA epicardial adipose tissue[64]
Longer AF duration[7]	Lack of AF termination[61]	
Hypertension[7]	Lack of SVC isolation[7]	
Nonparoxysmal AF[7]		
Higher CHA2DS2VASC score[60]		

Abbreviations: LV, left ventricular; SVC, superior vena cava.

who underwent redo ablations, PV reconnections were common and found in 81% of the patients and 93% underwent non-PV ablations including posterior wall isolation, cavotricuspid isthmus line, roof lines, superior vena cava ablation, and septal to right PVs. Following redo ablation, 75% of the patients were arrhythmia free at 17 months.[33]

Strategies for Repeat Ablation

Our mechanistic understanding of AF and therefore our ablation strategy is predicated on the following: AF is initiated by triggers, the most common of which are the PVs, and it is maintained by an electrically vulnerable atrial substrate. In cases of recurrence, our ablation strategy is focused on eliminating PV and extra PV triggers, and considering substrate modification guided by electroanatomic mapping.

PULMONARY VEIN REISOLATION

Elimination of AF triggers from the PVs by circumferential PVI is the primary strategy for AF ablation. Reconnected PVs are frequently encountered during redo ablations for recurrent AF. A meta-analysis of studies describing PV conduction in patients with and without AF recurrence showed that at least 1 PV was reconnected in 86% of patients with recurrence compared with 59% among patients without recurrence.[34] Lin and colleagues[35] identified reconnection of one or more PVs in more than 90% of the patients undergoing third or greater than third ablation procedure. The implication of finding reconnected veins during a redo procedure is ongoing triggers from the PVs. As such, our primary ablation strategy during reablation is identification and isolation of reconnected veins.

ABLATION OF NONPULMONARY VEIN TRIGGERS

In our practice, we routinely evaluate for the presence of non-PV triggers during initial and redo ablation procedures. Santangeli and colleagues[36] reported that non-PV triggers were present in 11% of the patients referred for ablation, regardless of duration and type of AF. Common sites of non-PV triggers include mitral annulus, fossa ovalis, Eustachian ridge, crista terminalis, and superior vena cava (**Fig. 2**).[37] Dixit and colleagues[38] compared the efficacy of ablation of non-PV triggers to substrate ablation in the form of CFAE ablation in addition to PVI in the RASTA study. In this RCT, non-PV trigger ablation strategy was found to be superior to CFAE ablation in terms of

freedom from atrial arrhythmias off AAD at 1 year after a single ablation procedure.[38]

Chronic PVI in patients with recurrent atrial arrhythmia has been rare in the past, but is happening more frequently as our ablation technology has improved. Sadek and colleagues[39] reported on patients undergoing redo ablation for AF and identified only 52 patients out of 1045 (5%) who had chronic PVI. Nearly half of these patients had atrial flutter or atrial tachycardia. Reablation strategies included non-PV trigger ablation, empiric trigger site ablation, provoked arrhythmia ablation, CFAE ablation, and linear ablation. In the absence of triggers, empiric ablation had less than 50% durable arrhythmia suppression.[39]

Thus, in our experience non-PV triggers represent an important target of ablation therapy. We favor the technique of eliciting and ablating triggers over empiric substrate ablation upfront for patients referred for redo ablation.

POSTERIOR WALL ISOLATION

The posterior wall has been postulated to be an AF trigger and play a role in maintenance of AF.[40] Subsequent studies have shown the feasibility of posterior wall isolation, but procedural success and impact on long-term outcomes have been variable.[41,42] In a more recent RCT, Lee and colleagues[43] reported that posterior wall isolation when added to PVI for the treatment of persistent AF did not result in improved clinical recurrence rates. In our practice, for patients with persistent AF we tend to proceed with posterior wall isolation, particularly if roof flutters are induced, or posterior wall triggers for AF are noted during electrophysiology study.

LEFT ATRIAL APPENDAGE ISOLATION

The LA appendage (LAA) has been recently identified as a potential source of non-PV trigger in patients referred for redo ablation. A retrospective study of patients undergoing redo catheter ablation for AF reported that nearly 30% of patients had LAA firing, and in 9% of the patients LAA was identified as the only trigger for AF. Complete isolation of the LAA was associated with lower recurrence of AF compared with focal lesions at the LAA and no ablation of the LAA.[44] This finding led to the BELIEF trial, which randomized 173 patients with long-standing persistent AF, all of whom had undergone prior ablation procedures to empirical LAA (LAA ablation) along with extensive ablation or extensive ablation alone. Extensive ablation included isolation of the PV antrum, posterior wall, anterior LA septum, and the LA roof.

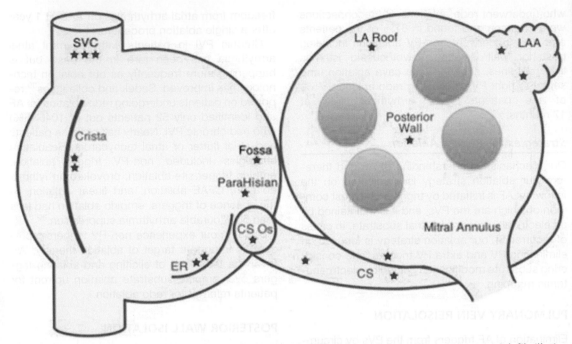

Fig. 2. Common sites of nonpulmonary vein triggers identified in patients with recurrent atrial fibrillation despite chronic pulmonary vein isolation. Red stars denote anatomic sites of nonpulmonary vein triggers for atrial fibrillation. CS; coronary sinus; ER, Eustacean ridge; LAA, left atrial appendage; SVC, superior vena cava. (*From* Sadek MM, Maeda S, Chik W et al. Recurrent atrial arrhythmias in the setting of chronic pulmonary vein isolation. Heart Rhythm 2016;13:2174-2180; with permission.)

At 12-month follow-up, 56% of the patients in the LAA isolation arm compared with 28% of patients in the extensive ablation alone arm were free of recurrent arrhythmias.[45] Despite the promising outcomes seen with LAA isolation, the benefits of sinus rhythm need to be weighed against the higher risk of stroke, which results from altered blood flow and stasis in the isolated LAA. Therapeutic anticoagulation is imperative in these patients and endovascular or surgical LAA occlusion therapies maybe required to mitigate the risk for stroke in patients with LAA isolation who are not candidates for anticoagulation, or who are at higher risk of thrombus formation despite anticoagulation. Other groups have found an alarming incidence of late thromboembolic complications despite continued anticoagulation.[46] This has led to the suggestion that LAA occlusion devices may be critical to the management of patients after LAA isolation, but this concept has not been tested in trials.

SUBSTRATE-BASED ABLATION

Elimination of PV and non-PV triggers may still be inadequate to treat recurrent AF, particularly in persistent AF, where abnormalities in atrial substrate may be dominant mechanism of AF maintenance. Importantly, none of these techniques were

endorsed in the recent AF ablation consensus document, based on insufficient or conflicting data on most "adjuvant" ablation strategies.[3] Multiple nonrandomized and small randomized studies had shown benefit for an empiric substrate–based approach, primarily linear lesions in the LA and/or elimination of CFAEs, in reducing AF recurrence.[47–50] The largest study to date (the STAR-AF II trial), however, randomized patients with persistent AF to PVI alone versus CFAE ablation or linear ablation across the LA roof and mitral valve isthmus in addition to PVI. At 18-month follow-up, there was no significant difference in freedom from arrhythmia recurrence after a single procedure between the groups.[51] In light of these data, in the absence of triggers or induction of atrial flutter or tachycardias during trigger protocol, we tend not to do empiric substrate ablation.

SUMMARY

As the understanding of mechanisms of AF evolves and the tools and techniques used in ablation improve, recurrence rates will improve. Hutchinson and colleagues[52] demonstrated that use of steerable introducers, high-frequency jet ventilation, and three-dimensional image integration were associated with more favorable 1-year freedom from AF compared with patients who underwent ablation without these techniques. The long-term outcomes in the current era of AF ablation marked by the use of contact sensing catheters, high-resolution mapping for atrial flutters, techniques such as high-power short-duration ablation lesions, and alternate sources of energy delivery (pulsed field ablation) remain to be seen.

Recurrent AF after RF ablation is common, with up to 50% of patients experiencing recurrence within 3 months. Early and multiple recurrences are harbingers of late recurrence within 1 year, which occurs in 20% to 50% of the patients, with persistent AF patients experiencing worse outcomes. Although there is no clear consensus regarding patient selection and timing of redo ablation, we refer symptomatic patients with multiple recurrences and persistent AF for redo ablation. Reisolation of the frequently encountered reconnected PVs and ablation of non-PV triggers is our primary ablation strategy for recurrent AF. In addition to repeat ablation, we recommend aggressive lifestyle modifications including weight loss, treatment of sleep-disordered breathing, and management of comorbid conditions for durable maintenance of sinus rhythm.

DISCLOSURE

The authors have nothing to disclose.

REFERENCES

1. Haissaguerre M, Jais P, Shah DC, et al. Spontaneous initiation of atrial fibrillation by ectopic beats originating in the pulmonary veins. N Engl J Med 1998;339:659–66.
2. Andrade JG, Khairy P, Verma A, et al. Early recurrence of atrial tachyarrhythmias following radiofrequency catheter ablation of atrial fibrillation. Pacing Clin Electrophysiol 2012;35:106–16.
3. Calkins H, Hindricks G, Cappato R, et al. 2017 HRS/EHRA/ECAS/APHRS/SOLAECE expert consensus statement on catheter and surgical ablation of atrial fibrillation: executive summary. Heart Rhythm 2017;14:e445–94.
4. Lee SH, Tai CT, Hsieh MH, et al. Predictors of early and late recurrence of atrial fibrillation after catheter ablation of paroxysmal atrial fibrillation. J Interv Card Electrophysiol 2004;10:221–6.
5. Andrade JG, Macle L, Khairy P, et al. Incidence and significance of early recurrences associated with different ablation strategies for AF: a STAR-AF substudy. J Cardiovasc Electrophysiol 2012;23:1295–301.
6. Liu J, Fang PH, Hou Y, et al. The value of transtelephonic electrocardiogram monitoring system during the "Blanking Period" after ablation of atrial fibrillation. J Electrocardiol 2010;43:667–72.
7. Themistoclakis S, Schweikert RA, Saliba WI, et al. Clinical predictors and relationship between early and late atrial tachyarrhythmias after pulmonary vein antrum isolation. Heart Rhythm 2008;5:679–85.
8. Koyama T, Sekiguchi Y, Tada H, et al. Comparison of characteristics and significance of immediate versus early versus no recurrence of atrial fibrillation after catheter ablation. Am J Cardiol 2009;103:1249–54.
9. Liang JJ, Elafros MA, Chik WW, et al. Early recurrence of atrial arrhythmias following pulmonary vein antral isolation: timing and frequency of early recurrences predicts long-term ablation success. Heart Rhythm 2015;12:2461–8.
10. Gerstenfeld EP, Callans DJ, Dixit S, et al. Mechanisms of organized left atrial tachycardias occurring after pulmonary vein isolation. Circulation 2004;110:1351–7.
11. Nademanee K, McKenzie J, Kosar E, et al. A new approach for catheter ablation of atrial fibrillation: mapping of the electrophysiologic substrate. J Am Coll Cardiol 2004;43:2044–53.
12. Rostock T, Drewitz I, Steven D, et al. Characterization, mapping, and catheter ablation of recurrent atrial tachycardias after stepwise ablation of long-lasting persistent atrial fibrillation. Circ Arrhythm Electrophysiol 2010;3:160–9.
13. Estner HL, Hessling G, Biegler R, et al. Complex fractionated atrial electrogram or linear ablation in patients with persistent atrial fibrillation: a prospective randomized study. Pacing Clin Electrophysiol 2011;34:939–48.
14. Wechselberger S, Kronborg M, Huo Y, et al. Continuous monitoring after atrial fibrillation ablation: the LINQ AF study. Europace 2018;20:f312–20.
15. Roux JF, Zado E, Callans DJ, et al. Antiarrhythmics after ablation of atrial fibrillation (5A study). Circulation 2009;120:1036–40.
16. Leong-Sit P, Roux JF, Zado E, et al. Antiarrhythmics after ablation of atrial fibrillation (5A study): six-month follow-up study. Circ Arrhythm Electrophysiol 2011;4:11–4.
17. Darkner S, Chen X, Hansen J, et al. Recurrence of arrhythmia following short-term oral AMIOdarone after CATheter ablation for atrial fibrillation: a double-blind, randomized, placebo-controlled study (AMIO-CAT trial). Eur Heart J 2014;35:3356–64.
18. Kaitani K, Inoue K, Kobori A, et al. Efficacy of antiarrhythmic drugs short-term use after catheter ablation for atrial fibrillation (EAST-AF) trial. Eur Heart J 2016;37:610–8.
19. Goldenberg GR, Burd D, Lodzinski P, et al. Antiarrhythmic therapy as an adjuvant to promote post pulmonary vein isolation success: a meta-analysis. J Interv Card Electrophysiol 2016;47:171–6.

20. Koyama T, Tada H, Sekiguchi Y, et al. Prevention of atrial fibrillation recurrence with corticosteroids after radiofrequency catheter ablation: a randomized controlled trial. J Am Coll Cardiol 2010;56:1463–72.

21. Kim YR, Nam GB, Han S, et al. Effect of short-term steroid therapy on early recurrence during the blanking period after catheter ablation of atrial fibrillation. Circ Arrhythm Electrophysiol 2015;8:1366–72.

22. Iskandar S, Reddy M, Afzal MR, et al. Use of oral steroid and its effects on atrial fibrillation recurrence and inflammatory cytokines post ablation. The steroid AF study. J Atr Fibrillation 2017;9:1604.

23. Deftereos S, Giannopoulos G, Kossyvakis C, et al. Colchicine for prevention of early atrial fibrillation recurrence after pulmonary vein isolation: a randomized controlled study. J Am Coll Cardiol 2012;60: 1790–6.

24. Deftereos S, Giannopoulos G, Efremidis M, et al. Colchicine for prevention of atrial fibrillation recurrence after pulmonary vein isolation: mid-term efficacy and effect on quality of life. Heart Rhythm 2014;11:620–8.

25. Pathak RK, Middeldorp ME, Lau DH, et al. Aggressive risk factor reduction study for atrial fibrillation and implications for the outcome of ablation: the ARREST-AF cohort study. J Am Coll Cardiol 2014; 64:2222–31.

26. Pathak RK, Middeldorp ME, Meredith M, et al. Long-term effect of goal-directed weight management in an atrial fibrillation cohort: a long-term follow-up study (LEGACY). J Am Coll Cardiol 2015;65: 2159–69.

27. Pathak RK, Elliott A, Middeldorp ME, et al. Impact of CARDIOrespiratory FITness on arrhythmia recurrence in obese individuals with atrial fibrillation: the CARDIO-FIT study. J Am Coll Cardiol 2015;66: 985–96.

28. Mohanty S, Mohanty P, DI Biase L, et al. Long-term outcome of catheter ablation in atrial fibrillation patients with coexistent metabolic syndrome and obstructive sleep apnea: impact of repeat procedures versus lifestyle changes. J Cardiovasc Electrophysiol 2014;25:930–8.

29. Das M, Wynn GJ, Morgan M, et al. Recurrence of atrial tachyarrhythmia during the second month of the blanking period is associated with more extensive pulmonary vein reconnection at repeat electrophysiology study. Circ Arrhythm Electrophysiol 2015;8:846–52.

30. Lellouche N, Jais P, Nault I, et al. Early recurrences after atrial fibrillation ablation: prognostic value and effect of early reablation. J Cardiovasc Electrophysiol 2008;19:599–605.

31. Tzou WS, Marchlinski FE, Zado ES, et al. Long-term outcome after successful catheter ablation of atrial fibrillation. Circ Arrhythm Electrophysiol 2010;3: 237–42.

32. Ganesan AN, Shipp NJ, Brooks AG, et al. Long-term outcomes of catheter ablation of atrial fibrillation: a systematic review and meta-analysis. J Am Heart Assoc 2013;2:e004549.

33. Shah S, Barakat AF, Saliba WI, et al. Recurrent atrial fibrillation after initial long-term ablation success: electrophysiological findings and outcomes of repeat ablation procedures. Circ Arrhythm Electrophysiol 2018;11:e005785.

34. Nery PB, Belliveau D, Nair GM, et al. Relationship between pulmonary vein reconnection and atrial fibrillation recurrence: a systematic review and meta-analysis. JACC Clin Electrophysiol 2016;2: 474–83.

35. Lin D, Santangeli P, Zado ES, et al. Electrophysiologic findings and long-term outcomes in patients undergoing third or more catheter ablation procedures for atrial fibrillation. J Cardiovasc Electrophysiol 2015;26:371–7.

36. Santangeli P, Zado ES, Hutchinson MD, et al. Prevalence and distribution of focal triggers in persistent and long-standing persistent atrial fibrillation. Heart Rhythm 2016;13:374–82.

37. Dixit S, Gerstenfeld EP, Ratcliffe SJ, et al. Single procedure efficacy of isolating all versus arrhythmogenic pulmonary veins on long-term control of atrial fibrillation: a prospective randomized study. Heart Rhythm 2008;5:174–81.

38. Dixit S, Marchlinski FE, Lin D, et al. Randomized ablation strategies for the treatment of persistent atrial fibrillation: RASTA study. Circ Arrhythm Electrophysiol 2012;5:287–94.

39. Sadek MM, Maeda S, Chik W, et al. Recurrent atrial arrhythmias in the setting of chronic pulmonary vein isolation. Heart Rhythm 2016;13:2174–80.

40. Kalifa J, Tanaka K, Zaitsev AV, et al. Mechanisms of wave fractionation at boundaries of high-frequency excitation in the posterior left atrium of the isolated sheep heart during atrial fibrillation. Circulation 2006;113:626–33.

41. Kumagai K, Muraoka S, Mitsutake C, et al. A new approach for complete isolation of the posterior left atrium including pulmonary veins for atrial fibrillation. J Cardiovasc Electrophysiol 2007;18:1047–52.

42. Kumar P, Bamimore AM, Schwartz JD, et al. Challenges and outcomes of posterior wall isolation for ablation of atrial fibrillation. J Am Heart Assoc 2016;5 [pii:e003885].

43. Lee JM, Shim J, Park J, et al. The electrical isolation of the left atrial posterior wall in catheter ablation of persistent atrial fibrillation. JACC Clin Electrophysiol 2019;5:1253–61.

44. Di Biase L, Burkhardt JD, Mohanty P, et al. Left atrial appendage: an underrecognized trigger site of atrial fibrillation. Circulation 2010;122:109–18.

45. Di Biase L, Burkhardt JD, Mohanty P, et al. Left atrial appendage isolation in patients with longstanding

persistent AF undergoing catheter ablation: BELIEF trial. J Am Coll Cardiol 2016;68:1929–40.

46. Heeger CH, Rillig A, Geisler D, et al. Left atrial appendage isolation in patients not responding to pulmonary vein isolation. Circulation 2019;139: 712–5.

47. Jais P, Hocini M, Hsu LF, et al. Technique and results of linear ablation at the mitral isthmus. Circulation 2004;110:2996–3002.

48. Knecht S, Hocini M, Wright M, et al. Left atrial linear lesions are required for successful treatment of persistent atrial fibrillation. Eur Heart J 2008;29: 2359–66.

49. Pak HN, Oh YS, Lim HE, et al. Comparison of voltage map-guided left atrial anterior wall ablation versus left lateral mitral isthmus ablation in patients with persistent atrial fibrillation. Heart Rhythm 2011; 8:199–206.

50. Willems S, Klemm H, Rostock T, et al. Substrate modification combined with pulmonary vein isolation improves outcome of catheter ablation in patients with persistent atrial fibrillation: a prospective randomized comparison. Eur Heart J 2006;27:2871–8.

51. Verma A, Jiang CY, Betts TR, et al. Approaches to catheter ablation for persistent atrial fibrillation. N Engl J Med 2015;372:1812–22.

52. Hutchinson MD, Garcia FC, Mandel JE, et al. Efforts to enhance catheter stability improve atrial fibrillation ablation outcome. Heart Rhythm 2013;10:347–53.

53. Oral H, Knight BP, Ozaydin M, et al. Clinical significance of early recurrences of atrial fibrillation after pulmonary vein isolation. J Am Coll Cardiol 2002; 40:100–4.

54. Della Bella P, Riva S, Fassini G, et al. Long-term follow-up after radiofrequency catheter ablation of atrial fibrillation: role of the acute procedure outcome and of the clinical presentation. Europace 2005;7:95–103.

55. Bertaglia E, Stabile G, Senatore G, et al. Predictive value of early atrial tachyarrhythmias recurrence after circumferential anatomical pulmonary vein ablation. Pacing Clin Electrophysiol 2005;28:366–71.

56. Richter B, Gwechenberger M, Socas A, et al. Frequency of recurrence of atrial fibrillation within 48

hours after ablation and its impact on long-term outcome. Am J Cardiol 2008;101:843–7.

57. Arya A, Hindricks G, Sommer P, et al. Long-term results and the predictors of outcome of catheter ablation of atrial fibrillation using steerable sheath catheter navigation after single procedure in 674 patients. Europace 2010;12:173–80.

58. Choi JI, Pak HN, Park JS, et al. Clinical significance of early recurrences of atrial tachycardia after atrial fibrillation ablation. J Cardiovasc Electrophysiol 2010;21:1331–7.

59. Verma A, Mantovan R, Macle L, et al. Substrate and trigger ablation for reduction of atrial fibrillation (STAR AF): a randomized, multicentre, international trial. Eur Heart J 2010;31:1344–56.

60. Kornej J, Hindricks G, Kosiuk J, et al. Comparison of CHADS2, R2CHADS2, and CHA2DS2-VASc scores for the prediction of rhythm outcomes after catheter ablation of atrial fibrillation: the Leipzig Heart Center AF ablation registry. Circ Arrhythm Electrophysiol 2014;7:281–7.

61. Li XP, Dong JZ, Liu XP, et al. Predictive value of early recurrence and delayed cure after catheter ablation for patients with chronic atrial fibrillation. Circ J 2008; 72:1125–9.

62. Moon J, Lee HJ, Kim JY, et al. Prognostic implications of right and left atrial enlargement after radiofrequency catheter ablation in patients with nonvalvular atrial fibrillation. Korean Circ J 2015;45: 301–9.

63. Kosiuk J, Breithardt OA, Bode K, et al. The predictive value of echocardiographic parameters associated with left ventricular diastolic dysfunction on short- and long-term outcomes of catheter ablation of atrial fibrillation. Europace 2014;16:1168–74.

64. Masuda M, Mizuno H, Enchi Y, et al. Abundant epicardial adipose tissue surrounding the left atrium predicts early rather than late recurrence of atrial fibrillation after catheter ablation. J Interv Card Electrophysiol 2015;44:31–7.

65. Joshi S, Choi AD, Kamath GS, et al. Prevalence, predictors, and prognosis of atrial fibrillation early after pulmonary vein isolation: findings from 3 months of continuous automatic ECG loop recordings. J Cardiovasc Electrophysiol 2009;20:1089–94.

Recurrent Atrial Fibrillation After Cryoballoon Ablation
What to Expect!

Arash Aryana, MD, PhD, FHRS[a],*, Gian-Battista Chierchia, MD, PhD[b],
Carlo de Asmundis, MD, PhD[b]

KEYWORDS

- Catheter ablation • Atrial fibrillation • Cryoballoon • Pulmonary vein isolation • Recurrence

KEY POINTS

- Atrial fibrillation (AF) can recur in patients following cryoballoon ablation due a variety of causes.
- In some, this may be a consequence of pulmonary vein (PV) reconnection, which may be effectively addressed by performing repeat catheter ablation to achieve optimal, antral bilateral PV isolation (PVI).
- In others, AF recurrence may manifest in presence of bilateral antral PVI.
- In such circumstances, one may elect to pursue catheter ablation of AF triggers, if present, or alternatively proceed with empiric posterior left atrial wall ablation and isolation.
- Although traditionally, point-by-point radiofrequency ablation has been used for this, cryoballoon ablation, itself, can also be used for ablation/isolation of certain anatomic structures, such as the superior vena cava, the left atrial appendage, and even the posterior left atrial wall with suitable outcomes.

Cryoballoon ablation has emerged as an effective strategy for the treatment of atrial fibrillation (AF).[1,2] Cryoballoon is designed to facilitate pulmonary vein isolation (PVI), which is considered the cornerstone and the primary goal of catheter ablation of AF.[3] The technique typically involves a single-shot approach by placing the balloon at the pulmonary vein (PV) ostia/antra, guided by PV occlusion. There are certain practical and theoretic advantages to cryoballoon ablation that include reduced pain and discomfort during ablation, improved catheter stability as a result of cryoadhesion between the tissue and the catheter, diminished risk of thrombosis due to decreased activation of platelets and coagulation cascade, uniform tissue necrosis due to lack of

vascular and endothelial disruption, preservation of connective tissue matrix, ability to rapidly create circumferential, contiguous lesions, and avoidance of steam pop.[4,5] In addition, the relative simplicity and gentle learning curve associated with this approach coupled with a consistently enhanced procedural workflow and efficiency have led to widespread adoption of this technology in clinical practice. Although some studies have shown a reduction in the incidence of mid-term[6] and long-term[7] AF recurrence following catheter ablation using the cryoballoon versus point-by-point radiofrequency, these findings have not been observed with the introduction of force-sensing radiofrequency ablation.[8,9] Nevertheless, AF recurrence is observed in up

[a] Mercy General Hospital and Dignity Health Heart and Vascular Institute, Suite #350, 3941 J Street, Sacramento, CA 95819, USA; [b] Heart Rhythm Management Center, UZ Brussel–VUB, Brussels, Belgium
* Corresponding author. Cardiovascular Services, Mercy General Hospital and Dignity Health Heart and Vascular Institute, 3941 J Street, Suite #350, Sacramento, CA 95819, USA.
E-mail address: a_aryana@outlook.com

Card Electrophysiol Clin 12 (2020) 199–208
https://doi.org/10.1016/j.ccep.2020.02.002
1877-9182/20/© 2020 Elsevier Inc. All rights reserved.

to 20% to 30% of paroxysmal and 40% to 60% of nonparoxysmal forms of AF during long-term follow-up.[10,11] In this article, we examine the common etiologies for AF recurrence following cryoballoon ablation of AF and methodologies for its treatment.

ATRIAL FIBRILLATION RECURRENCE

Most AF recurrences are commonly encountered within the first year following cryoballoon ablation. In particular, early recurrence within the initial 3 months following the procedure strongly predicts late recurrence.[12] On the other hand, very late recurrences (>1 year postablation) are often overlooked due to sparse follow-up and also the asymptomatic nature of arrhythmia recurrences following catheter ablation in some patients.[13]

Several studies have investigated the clinical predictors of AF recurrence following catheter ablation and have identified certain characteristics, such as left atrial size, hypertension, chronic kidney disease, and untreated sleep apnea as significant predictors.[14–17] However, PV reconnection primarily due to the failure to achieve complete and continuous transmural lesions remains an important etiology in patients who present with recurrent AF.[18,19] Having said that, it still remains clear whether PV reconnection is the only cause of arrhythmia recurrence in patients following AF ablation. Until now, only 2 small studies have investigated this question. Willems and colleagues[20] performed PVI in 64 patients with paroxysmal AF. After 3 months, nearly two-thirds of the patients underwent a repeat procedure irrespective of arrhythmia recurrence. Overall, PV reconnection was observed in 43% of the

PVs, whereas the number of reconnected PVs was significantly higher in those with versus without AF recurrence (1 vs 2 PVs; $P = .006$). On the other hand, in patients with durable PVI after 3 months, no symptoms or documentation of arrhythmia recurrence were noted. In another study, by Ouyang and colleagues,[21] 7 patients without arrhythmia recurrence underwent a repeat procedure to investigate the status of their PVs following an initial PVI procedure. In these patients, all PVs showed durable isolation as compared with those with arrhythmia recurrence. As such, the results from these studies underscore the importance of durable PVI. As such, the author believes it is valuable to offer patients with recurrent symptomatic AF a repeat procedure to further investigate for this and other triggers for AF to maximize the outcome of AF ablation. In this article, we examine the various scenarios and the respective approach during a repeat electrophysiology study and catheter ablation.

ATRIAL FIBRILLATION RECURRENCE IN PRESENCE OF PULMONARY VEIN RECONNECTION

PV reconnection or incomplete (distal, nonantral) isolation (**Fig. 1**A) is believed to account for one of the key mechanisms in recurrence of AF following catheter ablation.[20,21] Although the pathophysiologic mechanisms underlying PV reconnection have not been clearly elucidated, recovery of tissue conduction following a transient phase of reversible tissue injury along with inflammation/edema has been proposed as the main process underlying PV reconnection. Kowalski and colleagues[22] reported on the histopathologic

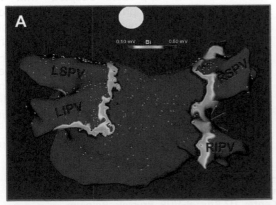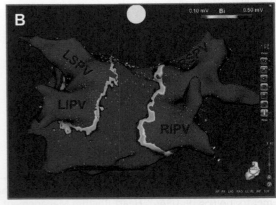

Fig. 1. Three-dimensional electroanatomic maps (voltage cutoff: 0.1–0.5 mV) created in 2 patients with recurrent AF following prior cryoballoon ablation. In one patient (*A*), the right PVs have not been effectively isolated. In the other patient (*B*), cryoballoon ablation has resulted in bilateral PVI at an acceptably proximal level. LIPV, left inferior pulmonary vein; LSPV, left superior pulmonary vein; RIPV, right inferior pulmonary vein; RSPV, right superior pulmonary vein.

and electrophysiologic findings in patients with recurrent AF following PVI performed during surgical Maze procedures. These investigators collected full-thickness PV antral surgical biopsy specimens where an endocardial scar was visible. They make an observation that presence of conduction block did not consistently correlate with transmural lesions at histopathologic analysis. In addition, these investigators found histopathologic findings consistent with reversible cellular injury up to 3 years after an index PVI. The latter may explain the occurrence of late PV reconnection.

Level of Pulmonary Vein Isolation

Cryoballoon ablation has been found to be an effective tool for PVI. As such, lesions created using the second-generation cryoballoon are typically large[23] and durable.[24] However, the level of PVI (ostial vs antral) using cryoballoon ablation has been the subject of controversy. Reddy and colleagues[23] were the first to investigate the level of PVI achieved using the cryoballoon. In their study, these investigators examined the precise location of ablation lesions created using a 23-mm first-generation cryoballoon (Arctic Front; Medtronic, Inc, Minneapolis, MN) in a cohort of patients using 3-dimensional electroanatomic mapping. They found that electrical isolation had occurred predominantly at the level of the PV ostia, whereas the PV antral tissue was left largely intact. In a subsequent study, Chierchia and colleagues[25] also evaluated the extent and level of PVI using both the 23-mm and the 28-mm first-generation cryoballoons. They noted that PVI had occurred more proximally using the 28-mm cryoballoon resulting in significantly larger areas of atrial tissue ablation ($40.2\% \pm 3.9\%$), as compared with the 23-mm balloon ($20.7\% \pm 2.8\%$). Most recently, Kenigsberg and colleagues[26] reported on a more contemporary experience using the 28-mm second-generation cryoballoon (Arctic Front Advance; Medtronic, Inc). The investigators found that the level of PVI was indeed much wider and more antral than previously thought. Furthermore, the investigators noticed partial isolation and debulking of the posterior left atrial wall by nearly 70% in a cohort of patients with paroxysmal AF and mild-to-moderate left atrial enlargement.

Along these lines, a recent study[27] comparing lesion characteristics and outcomes associated with PVI using the hot balloon versus the cryoballoon, found that lesions created using the latter were significantly larger (38 ± 12 cm^2 vs 24 ± 8 cm^2). Consequently, fewer instances of touch-up radiofrequency ablation were required with cryoballoon (31% vs 53%). Perrotta and colleagues,[28] who studied the size of left atrial isolation

following AF ablation using the laser versus the cryoballoon, had similar observations. The investigators found that total (42 ± 15 cm^2 vs 57 ± 14 cm^2; $P = .002$) and antral ($54 \pm 10\%$ vs $65 \pm 8\%$; $P = .001$) surface area isolation was greater using the cryoballoon. Another recent study[29] found that the low-voltage areas attained using the cryoballoon are significantly greater in size and the unexcitable tissue along the ablation lines are much wider than those created with point-by-point radiofrequency ablation. In addition, our group has previously illustrated that the incidence of PV reconnection is overall lower using the cryoballoon versus nonforce sensing point-by-point radiofrequency ablation (18.8% vs 34.6%; $P<.001$).[30] However, cryoballoon ablation was associated with a higher incidence of inferior and left common PV reconnection during follow-up electrophysiology study/catheter ablation. Other investigators[31] have identified the left superior PV, particularly the tissue along the "thicker" left atrial appendage (LAA) ridge as a common site of reconnection possibly due to a suboptimal transmural cryoablation at this site.

As such, at repeat electrophysiology study in a patient with recurrent AF following prior catheter ablation, the principal approach should always include demonstration and completion of bilateral antral PVI. Some experts have argued to use tools other than the cryoballoon (eg, focal radiofrequency) for completion of PVI in such cases. Although this seems reasonable, the authors believe the decision should be made on a case-by-case basis and guided by individual and anatomic variables. For instance, although an operator may choose to use point-by-point radiofrequency ablation for re-isolation of a large and anatomically challenging common PV or a reconnected inferior PV with marked tortuosity/acute takeoff, she or he may choose to re-ablate a reconnected left PV with an anatomy suited for cryoballoon ablation using by a tailored approach. That is, recent data suggest that PVI using the cryoballoon guided by a prespecified dosing algorithm may be associated with improved efficacy and safety.[32,33] Prior studies have demonstrated the utility of certain procedural (eg, time-to-PVI) and biophysical variables (ie, interval thaw time) in guiding cryoballoon applications.[34,35] Hence, cryoballoon ablation performed guided by such metrics can significantly enhance the long-term durability of PVI.[34]

ATRIAL FIBRILLATION RECURRENCE IN PRESENCE OF ANTRAL PULMONARY VEIN ISOLATION

Despite durable PVI following catheter ablation, a subset of patients still continue to experience recurrent AF (**Fig. 1**B). In a study by Dukkipati and colleagues,[36] AF recurrence was noted in 29% of the patients at 1 year in the face of proven PVI. The reasons underlying this lack of inadequate response to PVI remain unclear. As such, there is no consensus on the approach to management of patients with recurrent AF following prior ablation at electrophysiology study who are found to have durable antral PVI. However, there is evidence in support for several types of ablative strategies.

Ablation of Atrial Fibrillation Triggers

The incremental value of additional substrate modification with linear, rotor, or complex fractionated atrial electrogram ablation remains unproven.[37–41] Alternatively, Narayan and colleagues[40] described a computational mapping technique capable of identifying localized AF sources that may correspond to organized reentrant circuits (ie, rotors) or focal impulses that have been reported in animal models of AF. The potential benefit of ablation of these localized sources, known as focal impulses and rotor modulation (FIRM), has been tested against conventional ablation in a multicenter observational study including 92 patients with predominantly persistent AF.[42] Localized rotors or focal impulses were identified in 97% of patients, and ablation of these sites resulted in AF termination or slowing in 86%. At 9 months of follow-up, patients who received FIRM ablation were found to have higher freedom from recurrent AF as compared with conventional ablation (82% vs 45%; P<.001). However, these initial findings have not been reproducible.[43,44]

On the other hand, the occurrence of AF triggers outside of the PVs has been shown to play an important role at least in observational studies.[45–49] One approach to provoke latent non-PV triggers is to infuse high-dose isoproterenol (up to 20 µg/min) in conjunction with cardioversion of the induced AF. Typically, non-PV triggers cluster in specific regions, such as the coronary sinus, the inferior mitral annulus, the interatrial septum, particularly at the fossa ovalis/limbus region, the LAA, the Eustachian ridge, the crista terminalis region, and the superior vena cava (SVC).[37,50,51] Other sites identified as AF triggers include the persistent left SVC and its remnant, the ligament of Marshall.[52–55] Once a trigger has been identified, it should be eliminated using catheter ablation.[37,51] Having said that, in a recent randomized controlled trial, empiric ablation at these common origins of AF triggers did not improve clinical outcomes. Hence, such an approach is currently not recognized as a standard part of the initial ablative strategy in patients with AF.[37] Meanwhile, the optimal strategy to target non-PV triggers varies according to the site of origin. Although in many areas, focal ablation (typically radiofrequency) is sufficient to successfully abolish the triggers, elimination of triggers arising from the SVC or the LAA can be performed successfully through the use of radiofrequency or cryoballoon ablation.[50,56]

Superior Vena Cava Isolation

Because the SVC and/or a persistent left SVC (**Fig. 2**) represent a common site of non-PV triggers, performing isolation of these structures may improve the clinical outcomes in certain patients with AF.[57,58] Unlike the laser balloon,[59] a few studies have found SVC isolation using the cryoballoon to be safe and successful both clinically[60] and also in a canine model.[61] To perform this safely, the cryoapplication durations are typically reduced (90–150 seconds), as phrenic nerve injury serves as a major concern and limitation of such an approach.[61] The authors have experience with cryoballoon-guided SVC isolation (unpublished data). We have performed this approach in 24 consecutive patients with symptomatic AF and related triggers (54% with paroxysmal AF). The mean cryoapplication duration was

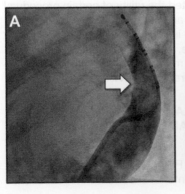
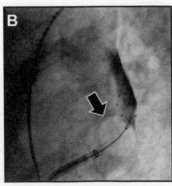

Fig. 2. Cryoballoon ablation of the persistent left SVC. (*A*) Angiography performed from within the coronary sinus in a left anterior oblique projection illustrating a persistent left SVC (*white arrow*). (*B*) Catheter ablation of this structure to achieve electrical isolation using the cryoballoon (*blue arrow*). (*From* Santoro et al. Second-Generation Cryoballoon Atrial Fibrillation Ablation in Patients With Persistent Left Superior Caval Vein. JACC Clin Electrophysiol 2019;5:590–598; with permission.)

117 ± 22 seconds. Although we observed 6 cases of transient phrenic nerve palsy (25%), persistent phrenic nerve palsy, defined as its presence through the end of the procedure, was avoided in all patients. However, one case of sinoatrial node dysfunction was encountered, prompting the insertion of a permanent pacemaker.

Left Atrial Appendage Isolation

Some investigators[50,62] have reported on the efficacy of isolation of the LAA as a potential source of AF, particularly in those with a clear, identifiable trigger.[63] Similar to SVC ablation, LAA isolation can be performed using point-by-point radiofrequency[50,62] or cryoballoon[64,65] ablation. Yorgun and colleagues[65] recently reported on their findings of cryoballoon-guided LAA isolation in addition to PVI in patients with symptomatic persistent AF, as compared with PVI alone. The

investigators found a higher incidence of freedom from recurrent arrhythmias at 1 year (86% vs 67%; P<.001). However, it is important to note that once LAA isolation has been achieved, the patient remains at a high risk for stroke and should therefore be committed to long-term, optimal, uninterrupted oral anticoagulation or LAA occlusion.[66]

Posterior Left Atrial Wall Isolation

Recent studies[67–69] have demonstrated the potential benefits associated with isolation of the posterior left atrial wall, which in fact shares a common embryologic origin with the PVs.[70] In addition, the posterior wall is also the site of several ganglionic plexi within the left atrium.[71] Moreover, a gross visual examination of the posterior wall and the orientation of the myofibrils also seem to suggest a direct continuity between this structure and the PV ostia (Fig. 3A), as does an anatomic

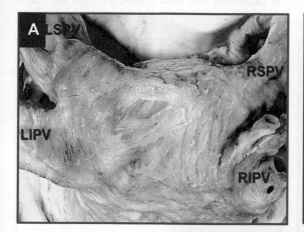
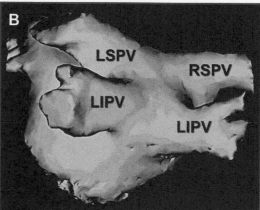
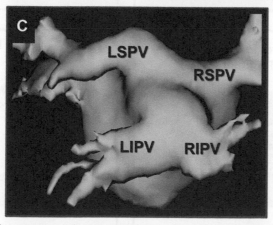

Fig. 3. Visual examination of the posterior left atrium and the pulmonary veins (PVs). (A) A gross anatomical examination highlighting the orientation of the myofibrils of the posterior left atrial wall and the PVs in the human. (B, C) Cardiac computed tomographic images from patients with AF illustrating variations in left atrial/PV anatomy. As seen, the precise boundaries between the posterior wall and the PVs remain obscure. Abbreviations: LIPV, denotes left inferior pulmonary vein; LSPV, left superior pulmonary vein; RIPV, right inferior pulmonary vein; and RSPV, right superior pulmonary vein. (Courtesy of André d'Avila, MD, PhD.)

assessment of certain left atrial morphologies by computed tomography (see **Fig. 3**B–C). In fact, in some cases it becomes difficult to distinguish the posterior wall from the PV antra and to determine the precise level at which to create PVI during AF ablation. Consequently, it is increasingly believed that an effective strategy for the treatment of patients at least with more advanced forms of AF or those with arrhythmia recurrence in presence of bilateral, antral PVI should involve this approach.[72] This is also supported by clinical and cellular data that suggest that in patients with AF the posterior wall exhibits significant conduction abnormalities, higher incidence of delayed after depolarizations, and larger late sodium and intracellular and sarcoplasmic reticulum Ca^{++} contents, but smaller inward rectifier potassium currents.[73,74]

To date, a variety of catheter-based techniques have been used to achieve posterior wall isolation (**Fig. 4**). One approach involves the "box" approach. Although feasible,[75] the theoretic

advantages of this strategy are in some cases offset by the challenges of creating uninterrupted, contiguous linear lesions.[76,77] In many instances, despite seemingly complete ablation linear lesions, pacing maneuvers within the "box" result in pace-capture and conduction to the left atrium.[78] Some experts have attributed this to the presence of epicardial connections/myofibrils. A second approach involves wide-area circumferential ablation, whereas a third strategy involves direct ablation of the posterior left atrial wall using either point-by-point radiofrequency[67] or the cryoballoon.[79,80] As previously mentioned, lesions created using the second-generation cryoballoon are generally large[23] and durable.[24] This renders this catheter a potentially attractive tool for performing posterior wall ablation. Moreover, some consider the cryoballoon overall a safer tool for this approach, particularly with regard to the esophagus. Although not required, the technique is facilitated and best guided through the use of

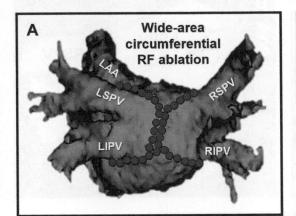
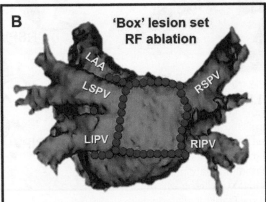
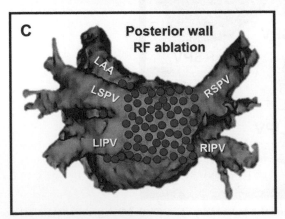
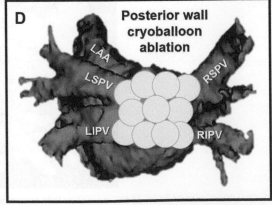

Fig. 4. Techniques for catheter ablation of the posterior left atrial wall. The strategies for isolating the posterior left atrial wall consist of wide-area circumferential ablation (*A*), the "box" lesion set (*B*) or direct posterior wall ablation using point-by-point radiofrequency (*C*) or the cryoballoon (*D*). LIPV, left inferior pulmonary vein; LSPV, left superior pulmonary vein; RF, radiofrequency; RIPV, right inferior pulmonary vein; RSPV, right superior pulmonary vein.

intracardiac echocardiography to allow direct visualization and integration into the 3-dimensional mapping system (CARTO; Biosense Webster, Inc, Irvine, CA).

Aryana and colleagues[79] recently performed a multicenter, retrospective study to analyze the outcomes of PVI in conjunction with direct posterior wall ablation/isolation using the second-generation cryoballoon in a cohort of patients with symptomatic persistent AF. The study found that posterior wall isolation using this method was feasible in approximately two-thirds of the patients without significant adverse events. Moreover, as compared with PVI alone, this approach was associated with marked reductions in recurrent AF/atrial arrhythmias at 1 year. In a subsequent study,[81] we reported on the long-term durability of posterior wall isolation using the same strategy in 61 (89%) of 69 patients who underwent this technique at 9 months of follow-up. Nonetheless, prospective randomized controlled trials are needed to validate the long-term outcomes of posterior wall ablation using the cryoballoon. A multicenter, multinational, prospective randomized controlled investigational device exemption trial is currently under way to specifically evaluate the long-term safety and efficacy of this approach.

In summary, AF can recur in patients following cryoballoon ablation due a variety of etiologies. In some, this may be effectively addressed by repeating optimal PVI to achieve complete, bilateral antral PV isolation. In others, AF recurrence may present despite bilateral antral PVI. In such circumstances, the operator may elect to pursue catheter ablation of AF triggers, if present, or alternatively proceed with posterior left atrial wall isolation. Traditionally, point-by-point radiofrequency ablation has been used for these purposes. However, cryoballoon ablation, itself, also can be used for ablation/isolation of certain structures such as the SVC, the LAA, and even the posterior wall with favorable safety and efficacy. Nonetheless, additional research is clearly needed to further characterize and distinguish the optimal tools and strategies for these patients.

DISCLOSURE

Drs A. Aryana, G. B. Chierchia and C. de Asmundis have received consulting fees, speaker honoraria and research grants from Medtronic, Biosense Webster, and Abbott.

REFERENCES

1. Packer DL, Kowal RC, Wheelan KR, et al, STOP AF Cryoablation Investigators. Cryoballoon ablation of pulmonary veins for paroxysmal atrial fibrillation: first results of the North American Arctic Front (STOP AF) pivotal trial. J Am Coll Cardiol 2013;61:1713–23.

2. Kuck KH, Brugada J, Fürnkranz A, et al, FIRE AND ICE Investigators. Cryoballoon or radiofrequency ablation for paroxysmal atrial fibrillation. N Engl J Med 2016;374:2235–45.

3. Haïssaguerre M, Jaïs P, Shah DC, et al. Spontaneous initiation of atrial fibrillation by ectopic beats originating in the pulmonary veins. N Engl J Med 1998;339:659–66.

4. Bredikis A, Wilber D. Factors that determine cryolesion formation and cryolesion characteristics. In: Bredikis A, Wilber D, editors. Cryoablation of cardiac arrhythmias. Philadelphia: Saunders; 2011. p. 22–39.

5. Khairy P, Chauvet P, Lehmann J, et al. Lower incidence of thrombus formation with cryoenergy versus radiofrequency catheter ablation. Circulation 2003;107:2045–50.

6. Aryana A, Singh SM, Kowalski M, et al. Acute and long-term outcomes of catheter ablation of atrial fibrillation using the second-generation cryoballoon versus open-irrigated radiofrequency: a multicenter experience. J Cardiovasc Electrophysiol 2015;26:832–9.

7. Galizia Brito V, Vecchio N, Tomas L, et al. Second generation cryoballoon vs. radiofrequency ablation in paroxysmal atrial fibrillation: outcomes beyond one-year follow-up. J Atr Fibrillation 2019;11:2147.

8. Andrade JG, Champagne J, Dubuc M, et al, CIRCA-DOSE Study Investigators. Cryoballoon or radiofrequency ablation for atrial fibrillation assessed by continuous monitoring: a randomized clinical trial. Circulation 2019. https://doi.org/10.1161/CIRCULATIONAHA.119.042622.

9. Jourda F, Providencia R, Marijon E, et al. Contact-force guided radiofrequency vs. second-generation balloon cryotherapy for pulmonary vein isolation in patients with paroxysmal atrial fibrillation—a prospective evaluation. Europace 2015;17:225–31.

10. Heeger CH, Wissner E, Knöll M, et al. Three-year clinical outcome after 2nd-generation cryoballoon-based pulmonary vein isolation for the treatment of paroxysmal and persistent atrial fibrillation – a 2-center experience. Circ J 2017;81:974–80.

11. Takarada K, Overeinder I, de Asmundis C, et al. Long-term outcome after second-generation cryoballoon ablation for paroxysmal atrial fibrillation – a 3-years follow-up. J Interv Card Electrophysiol 2017;49:93–100.

12. Kornej J, Schumacher K, Dinov B, et al. Prediction of electro-anatomical substrate and arrhythmia recurrences using APPLE, DR-FLASH and MB-LATER scores in patients with atrial fibrillation undergoing catheter ablation. Sci Rep 2018;8:12686.

13. Shah S, Barakat AF, Saliba WI, et al. Recurrent atrial fibrillation after initial long-term ablation success: electrophysiological findings and outcomes of repeat ablation procedures. Circ Arrhythm Electrophysiol 2018;11:e005785.

14. Njoku A, Kannabhiran M, Arora R, et al. Left atrial volume predicts atrial fibrillation recurrence after radiofrequency ablation: a meta-analysis. Europace 2018;20:33–42.

15. Lin KJ, Cho S, Tiwari N, et al. Impact of metabolic syndrome on the risk of atrial fibrillation recurrence after catheter ablation: systematic review and meta-analysis. J Interv Card Electrophysiol 2014; 39:211–23.

16. Li M, Liu T, Luo D, et al. Systematic review and meta-analysis of chronic kidney disease as predictor of atrial fibrillation recurrence following catheter ablation. Cardiol J 2014;21:89–95.

17. Goes CM, Falcochio PPNF, Drager LF. Strategies to manage obstructive sleep apnea to decrease the burden of atrial fibrillation. Expert Rev Cardiovasc Ther 2018;16:707–13.

18. Nilsson B, Chen X, Pehrson S, et al. Recurrence of pulmonary vein conduction and atrial fibrillation after pulmonary vein isolation for atrial fibrillation: a randomized trial of the ostial versus the extraostial ablation strategy. Am Heart J 2006;152:537.e1-8.

19. Van Belle Y, Janse P, Theuns D, et al. One year follow-up after cryoballoon isolation of the pulmonary veins in patients with paroxysmal atrial fibrillation. Europace 2008;10:1271–6.

20. Willems S, Steven D, Servatius H, et al. Persistence of pulmonary vein isolation after robotic remote-navigated ablation for atrial fibrillation and its relation to clinical outcome. J Cardiovasc Electrophysiol 2010;21:1079–84.

21. Ouyang F, Antz M, Ernst S, et al. Recovered pulmonary vein conduction as a dominant factor for recurrent atrial tachyarrhythmias after complete circular isolation of the pulmonary veins: lessons from double Lasso technique. Circulation 2005;111:127–35.

22. Kowalski M, Grimes MM, Perez FJ, et al. Histopathologic characterization of chronic radiofrequency ablation lesions for pulmonary vein isolation. J Am Coll Cardiol 2012;59:930–8.

23. Reddy VY, Neuzil P, d'Avila A, et al. Balloon catheter ablation to treat paroxysmal atrial fibrillation: what is the level of pulmonary venous isolation? Heart Rhythm 2008;5:353–60.

24. Reddy VY, Sediva L, Petru J, et al. Durability of pulmonary vein isolation with cryoballoon ablation: results from the SUstained PV Isolation with ARctic Front Advance (SUPIR) Study. J Cardiovasc Electrophysiol 2015;26:493–500.

25. Chierchia GB, de Asmundis C, Sorgente A, et al. Anatomical extent of pulmonary vein isolation after cryoballoon ablation for atrial fibrillation: comparison between the 23 and 28 mm balloons. J Cardiovasc Med (Hagerstown) 2011;12:162–6.

26. Kenigsberg DN, Martin N, Lim HW, et al. Quantification of the cryoablation zone demarcated by pre- and postprocedural electroanatomic mapping in patients with atrial fibrillation using the 28-mm second-generation cryoballoon. Heart Rhythm 2015;12:283–90.

27. Nagashima K, Okumura Y, Watanabe I, et al. Hot balloon versus cryoballoon ablation for atrial fibrillation: lesion characteristics and efficacy. Circ Arrhythm Electrophysiol 2018;11(5):e005861.

28. Perrotta L, Konstantinou A, Bordignon S, et al. What is the acute antral lesion size after pulmonary vein isolation using different balloon ablation technologies? Circ J 2017;81:172–9.

29. Okumura Y, Watanabe I, Iso K, et al. Mechanistic insights into durable pulmonary vein isolation achieved by second-generation cryoballoon ablation. J Atr Fibrillation 2017;9:18–24.

30. Aryana A, Singh SM, Mugnai G, et al. Pulmonary vein reconnection following catheter ablation of atrial fibrillation using the second-generation cryoballoon versus open-irrigated radiofrequency: results of a multicenter analysis. J Interv Card Electrophysiol 2016;47:341–8.

31. Shah S, Xu W, Adelstein E, et al. Characterization of pulmonary vein reconnection post cryoballoon ablation. Indian Pacing Electrophysiol J 2019;19:129–33.

32. Aryana A, Kenigsberg DN, Kowalski M, et al, CryoDOSING Investigators. Verification of a novel atrial fibrillation cryoablation dosing algorithm guided by time-to-pulmonary vein isolation: results from the cryo-DOSING study (Cryoballoon-ablation DOSING based on the assessment of time-to-effect and pulmonary vein isolation guidance). Heart Rhythm 2017;14:1319–25.

33. Chun KR, Stich M, Fürnkranz A, et al. Individualized cryoballoon energy pulmonary vein isolation guided by real-time pulmonary vein recordings, the randomized ICE-T trial. Heart Rhythm 2017;14:495–500.

34. Aryana A, Mugnai G, Singh SM, et al. Procedural and biophysical indicators of durable pulmonary vein isolation during cryoballoon ablation of atrial fibrillation. Heart Rhythm 2016;13:424–32.

35. Ghosh J, Martin A, Keech AC, et al. Balloon warming time is the strongest predictor of late pulmonary vein electrical reconnection following cryoballoon ablation for atrial fibrillation. Heart Rhythm 2013;10:1311–7.

36. Dukkipati SR, Neuzil P, Kautzner J, et al. The durability of pulmonary vein isolation using the visually guided laser balloon catheter: multicenter results of pulmonary vein remapping studies. Heart Rhythm 2012;9:919–25.

37. Dixit S, Marchlinski FE, Lin D, et al. Randomized ablation strategies for the treatment of persistent

atrial fibrillation: RASTA study. Circ Arrhythm Electro-physiol 2012;5:287–94.

38. Dixit S, Lin D, Frankel DS, et al. Catheter ablation for persistent atrial fibrillation: antral pulmonary vein isolation and elimination of nonpulmonary vein triggers are sufficient. Circ Arrhythm Electrophysiol 2012;5:1216–23.

39. Bai R, Di Biase L, Mohanty P, et al. Ablation of peri-mitral flutter following catheter ablation of atrial fibrillation: impact on outcomes from a randomized study (PROPOSE). J Cardiovasc Electrophysiol 2012;23: 137–44.

40. Skanes AC, Mandapati R, Berenfeld O, et al. Spatio-temporal periodicity during atrial fibrillation in the isolated sheep heart. Circulation 1998;98:1236–48.

41. Narayan SM, Krummen DE, Rappel WJ. Clinical mapping approach to diagnose electrical rotors and focal impulse sources for human atrial fibrillation. J Cardiovasc Electrophysiol 2012;23: 447–54.

42. Narayan SM, Krummen DE, Shivkumar K, et al. Treatment of atrial fibrillation by the ablation of localized sources: CONFIRM (conventional ablation for atrial fibrillation with or without focal impulse and rotor modulation) trial. J Am Coll Cardiol 2012;60: 628–36.

43. Buch E, Share M, Tung R, et al. Long-term clinical outcomes of focal impulse and rotor modulation for treatment of atrial fibrillation: a multicenter experience. Heart Rhythm 2016;13:636–41.

44. Benharash P, Buch E, Frank P, et al. Quantitative analysis of localized sources identified by focal impulse and rotor modulation mapping in atrial fibrillation. Circ Arrhythm Electrophysiol 2015;8:554–61.

45. Santangeli P, di Biase L, Pelargonio G, et al. Outcome of invasive electrophysiological procedures and gender: are males and females the same? J Cardiovasc Electrophysiol 2011;22:605–12.

46. Santangeli P, Di Biase L, Horton R, et al. Ablation of atrial fibrillation under therapeutic warfarin reduces periprocedural complications: evidence from a meta-analysis. Circ Arrhythm Electrophysiol 2012; 5:302–11.

47. Lakkireddy D, Nagarajan D, Di Biase L, et al. Radio-frequency ablation of atrial fibrillation in patients with mitral or aortic mechanical prosthetic valves: a feasibility, safety and efficacy study. Heart Rhythm 2011; 8:975–80.

48. Mohanty S, Mohanty P, Di Biase L, et al. Impact of metabolic syndrome on procedural outcomes in patients with atrial fibrillation undergoing catheter ablation. J Am Coll Cardiol 2012;59:1295–301.

49. Patel D, Mohanty P, Di Biase L, et al. Safety and efficacy of pulmonary vein antral isolation in patients with obstructive sleep apnea: the impact of continuous positive airway pressure. Circ Arrhythm Electrophysiol 2010;3:445–51.

50. Di Biase L, Burkhardt JD, Mohanty P, et al. Left atrial appendage: an underrecognized trigger site of atrial fibrillation. Circulation 2010;122:109–18.

51. Dixit S, Gerstenfeld EP, Ratcliffe SJ, et al. Single procedure efficacy of isolating all versus arrhythmogenic pulmonary veins on long-term control of atrial fibrillation: a prospective randomized study. Heart Rhythm 2008;5:174–81.

52. Hsu LF, Jaïs P, Keane D, et al. Atrial fibrillation originating from persistent left superior vena cava. Circulation 2004;109:828–32.

53. Elayi CS, Fahmy TS, Wazni OM, et al. Left superior vena cava isolation in patients undergoing pulmonary vein antrum isolation: impact on atrial fibrillation recurrence. Heart Rhythm 2006;3:1019–23.

54. Han S, Joung B, Scanavacca M, et al. Electrophysiological characteristics of the Marshall bundle in humans. Heart Rhythm 2010;7:786–93.

55. Valderrábano M, Chen HR, Sidhu J, et al. Retrograde ethanol infusion in the vein of Marshall: regional left atrial ablation, vagal denervation and feasibility in humans. Circ Arrhythm Electrophysiol 2009;2:50–6.

56. Di Biase L, Bai R, Mohanty P, et al. Atrial fibrillation triggers from the coronary sinus: comparison between isolation versus focal ablation. Heart Rhythm 2011;8(Suppl. 1):S78.

57. Arruda M, Mlcochova H, Prasad SK, et al. Electrical isolation of the superior vena cava: an adjunctive strategy to pulmonary vein antrum isolation improving the outcome of AF ablation. J Cardiovasc Electrophysiol 2007;18:1261–6.

58. Corrado A, Bonso A, Madalosso M, et al. Impact of systematic isolation of superior vena cava in addition to pulmonary vein antrum isolation on the outcome of paroxysmal, persistent, and permanent atrial fibrillation ablation: results from a randomized study. J Cardiovasc Electrophysiol 2010;21:1–5.

59. Arceluz MR, Cruz PF, Falconi E, et al. Electrical isolation of the superior vena cava by laser balloon ablation in patients with atrial fibrillation. J Interv Card Electrophysiol 2018;53:217–23.

60. Huang S, Pan B, Zou H, et al. Cryoballoon ablation for paroxysmal atrial fibrillation in a case of persistent left superior vena cava. BMC Cardiovasc Disord 2018;18:51.

61. Wei HQ, Li J, Sun Q, et al. Safety and efficacy of superior vena cava isolation using the second-generation cryoballoon ablation in a canine model. J Cardiol 2019;75(4):368–73.

62. Hocini M, Shah AJ, Nault I, et al. Localized reentry within the left atrial appendage: arrhythmogenic role in patients under-going ablation of persistent atrial fibrillation. Heart Rhythm 2011;8:1853–61.

63. Yorgun H, Canpolat U, Evranos B, et al. Entrapment of focal atrial tachycardia using cryoballoon ablation;Sinus rhythm in the left atrium and ongoing atrial

tachycardia in the left atrial appendage. Indian Pacing Electrophysiol J 2017;17:189–91.

64. Bordignon S, Chen S, Perrotta L, et al. Durability of cryoballoon left atrial appendage isolation: acute and invasive remapping electrophysiological findings. Pacing Clin Electrophysiol 2019;42:646–54.

65. Yorgun H, Canpolat U, Kocyigit D, et al. Left atrial appendage isolation in addition to pulmonary vein isolation in persistent atrial fibrillation: one-year clinical outcome after cryoballoon-based ablation. Europace 2017;19:758–68.

66. Di Biase L, Mohanty S, Trivedi C, et al. Stroke risk in patients with atrial fibrillation undergoing electrical isolation of the left atrial appendage. J Am Coll Cardiol 2019;74:1019–28.

67. Bai R, Di Biase L, Mohanty P, et al. Proven isolation of the pulmonary vein antrum with or without left atrial posterior wall isolation in patients with persistent atrial fibrillation. Heart Rhythm 2016;13:132–40.

68. He X, Zhou Y, Chen Y, et al. Left atrial posterior wall isolation reduces the recurrence of atrial fibrillation: a meta-analysis. J Interv Card Electrophysiol 2016; 46:267–74.

69. Gökoğlan Y, Mohanty S, Güneş MF, et al. Pulmonary vein antrum isolation in patients with paroxysmal atrial fibrillation: more than a decade of follow-up. Circ Arrhythm Electrophysiol 2016;9(5) [pii: e003660].

70. Bai R. Left atrial posterior wall isolation: the icing on the cake. J Interv Card Electrophysiol 2016;46: 199–201.

71. Po SS, Nakagawa H, Jackman WM. Localization of left atrial ganglionated plexi in patients with atrial fibrillation. J Cardiovasc Electrophysiol 2009;20: 1186–9.

72. Calkins H, Hindricks G, Cappato R, et al. 2017 HRS/EHRA/ECAS/APHRS/SOLAECE expert consensus statement on catheter and surgical ablation of atrial fibrillation. Heart Rhythm 2017;14:e275–444.

73. Markides V, Schilling RJ, Ho SY, et al. Characterization of left atrial activation in the intact human heart. Circulation 2003;107:733–9.

74. Suenari K, Chen YC, Kao YH, et al. Discrepant electrophysiological characteristics and calcium homeostasis of left atrial anterior and posterior myocytes. Basic Res Cardiol 2011;106:65–74.

75. Lim TW, Koay CH, See VA, et al. Single-ring posterior left atrial (box) isolation results in a different mode of recurrence compared with wide antral pulmonary vein isolation on long-term follow-up: longer atrial fibrillation-free survival time but similar survival time free of any atrial arrhythmia. Circ Arrhythm Electrophysiol 2012;5:968–77.

76. Reddy VY, Neuzil P, D'Avila A, et al. Isolating the posterior left atrium and pulmonary veins with a "box" lesion set: use of epicardial ablation to complete electrical isolation. J Cardiovasc Electrophysiol 2008;19:326–9.

77. Higuchi S, Sohara H, Nakamura Y, et al. Is it necessary to achieve a complete box isolation in the case of frequent esophageal temperature rises? Feasibility of shifting to a partial box isolation strategy for patients with non-paroxysmal atrial fibrillation. J Cardiovasc Electrophysiol 2016;27:897–904.

78. Kumar P, Bamimore AM, Schwartz JD, et al. Challenges and outcomes of posterior wall isolation for ablation of atrial fibrillation. J Am Heart Assoc 2016;5(9) [pii:e003885].

79. Aryana A, Baker JH, Espinosa Ginic MA, et al. Posterior wall isolation using the cryoballoon in conjunction with pulmonary vein ablation is superior to pulmonary vein isolation alone in patients with persistent atrial fibrillation: a multicenter experience. Heart Rhythm 2018;15:1121–9.

80. Nishimura T, Yamauchi Y, Aoyagi H, et al. The clinical impact of the left atrial posterior wall lesion formation by the cryoballoon application for persistent atrial fibrillation: feasibility and clinical implications. J Cardiovasc Electrophysiol 2019;30:805–14.

81. Aryana A, Baker JH, Espinosa MA, et al. Long-term durability of posterior wall isolation in conjunction with pulmonary vein ablation using the cryoballoon in patients with persistent atrial fibrillation: outcomes from a multicenter experience. Heart Rhythm 2019; 16(5):S19.

Recurrent Atrial Fibrillation with Isolated Pulmonary Veins: What to Do

Carola Gianni, MD[a],*, Alisara Anannab, MD[a,e],
Domenico G. Della Rocca, MD[a], Anu Salwan, MD[a], Bryan MacDonald, MD[a],
Angel Quintero Mayedo, MD[a], Sanghamitra Mohanty, MD[a,f],
Chintan Trivedi, MD[a], Luigi Di Biase, MD[a,g,h], Andrea Natale, MD[a,b,c,d]

KEYWORDS

- Atrial fibrillation ablation • Nonpulmonary vein triggers • Superior vena cava • Coronary sinus
- Left atrial posterior wall • Left atrial appendage

KEY POINTS

- When patients have symptomatic recurrent atrial tachyarrhythmias after 2 months following pulmonary vein antral isolation, a repeat ablation should be considered.
- In these patients, nonpulmonary vein triggers should be actively sought and ablated.
- In patients with nonparoxysmal atrial fibrillation or known higher prevalence of nonpulmonary vein triggers, empirical isolation of the superior vena cava, coronary sinus, and/or left atrial appendage might be performed.

Success rates after a single pulmonary vein antral isolation (PVAI) procedure are variable. They mainly depend on the type of atrial fibrillation (AF), presence of comorbidities, experience of the electrophysiologist performing the procedure, technology used, and duration/intensity of follow-up.[1] When patients have symptomatic recurrent atrial tachyarrhythmias after 2 months following PVAI, a repeat ablation should be considered.

Some patients, to varying degrees, have regain of pulmonary vein (PV) conduction and antral electrical activity; PV reisolation is therefore performed, including complete empirical posterior

wall (PW) isolation, if this was not performed at the time of the first procedure. Other patients might present with persistent isolated PVs and a silent antrum (ie, isolated PW). In these patients, PW isolation is extended, and non-PV triggers are actively sought and ablated. Moreover, in those with nonparoxysmal AF or a known higher prevalence of non-PV triggers (**Table 1**), empirical isolation of the superior vena cava (SVC), coronary sinus (CS), and/or left atrial appendage (LAA) might be performed.[2]

In this review, the authors focus on ablation of non-PV triggers, summarizing our current approach for their mapping and ablation.

a Texas Cardiac Arrhythmia Institute, St. David's Medical Center, Austin, TX, USA; b HCA National Medical Director of Cardiac Electrophysiology, USA; c Interventional Electrophysiology, Scripps Clinic, La Jolla, CA, USA; d MetroHealth Medical Center, Case Western Reserve University School of Medicine, Cleveland, OH, USA; e Electrophysiology Unit, Department of Cardiovascular Interventions, Central Chest Institute of Thailand, Nonthaburi, Thailand; f Dell Medical School, University of Texas, Austin, TX, USA; g Montefiore Medical Center, Albert Einstein College of Medicine, Bronx, NY, USA; h Department of Clinical and Experimental Medicine, University of Foggia, Foggia, Italy
* Corresponding author. Texas Cardiac Arrhythmia Institute, St. David's Medical Center, 3000 N. IH-35, Suite 720, Austin, TX 78705.
E-mail address: carola.gianni@gmail.com

Card Electrophysiol Clin 12 (2020) 209–217
https://doi.org/10.1016/j.ccep.2020.02.001
1877-9182/20/© 2020 Elsevier Inc. All rights reserved.

Table 1
Subset of patients with higher prevalence of nonpulmonary vein triggers

Patients with Higher Prevalence of Non-PV Triggers	
Nonparoxysmal AF	Low LVEF
Female gender	Severe LA scarring
Older age	Hypertrophic
Obesity	cardiomyopathy
Sleep apnea	Mechanical mitral valve
	Late recurrence post-PVAI in PAF

Abbreviations: LA, left atrium; LVEF, left ventricular ejection fraction; PAF, paroxysmal atrial fibrillation.
From Gianni C, Mohanty S, Trivedi C, Di Biase L, Natale A. Novel concepts and approaches in ablation of atrial fibrillation: the role of non-pulmonary vein triggers. *EP Eur.* 2018;20(10):1566-1576; with permission.

ABLATION OF NONPULMONARY VEIN TRIGGERS

Non-PV triggers are ectopic beats triggering AF, originating in areas other than the PVs. They usually cluster in specific regions such as the left atrial PW, other thoracic veins (SVC, CS, vein of Marshall), crista terminalis (CR), interatrial septum (IAS), and the LAA. These structures have myocardial cells that retain the ability to automatically depolarize or serve a substrate for micro-reentry due to their rapid conduction, thus serving as independent triggers for AF.[3,4]

Ablation of non-PV triggers can be empiric or performed after induction using high-dose isoproterenol (an infusion of 20–30 µg/min for 10–15 minutes, with concomitant adequate pressure support). For the latter approach, it is important that any antiarrhythmic drug is stopped at least 5 half-lives before the procedure, to minimize the chance of noninducibility. Mapping non-PV triggers is guided by multiple catheters positioned along both the right and left atrium (**Fig. 1**): a 10-pole circular mapping catheter (CMC) in the left superior PV recording the far-field LAA activity (to avoid mechanical ectopies), the ablation catheter in the right superior PV that records the far-field interatrial septum, and a 20-pole linear catheter with electrodes spanning from the SVC, right atrium/CR to the CS. When focal ectopic atrial activity is observed, their activation sequence is compared with that of sinus rhythm, allowing to quickly identify their area of origin:

- Beats originating from the right atrium: earliest activation in the proximal duo-decapolar catheter; the specific activation sequence varies depending on the site of origin, resembling that of sinus rhythm for ectopies originating from the SVC (see **Fig. 1**, green)
- Beats originating from the IAS area: both the CS and proximal duo-decapolar catheter are early, usually preceded by the far-field atrial activity recorded with the ablation catheter (see **Fig. 1**, magenta)
- Beats originating from the CS: earliest activation in the distal duo-decapolar catheter (see **Fig. 1**, blue)
- Beats originating from the LAA: far-field activity in the CMC is early, preceding that recorded in the distal CS (see **Fig. 1**, yellow)

For significant non-PV triggers (repetitive isolated premature atrial contractions [PACs], focal atrial tachycardias, or beats triggering AF/atrial flutter), a more detailed activation mapping can be performed in the area of origin. In general, non-PV trigger are targeted with focal ablation, exception being the triggers originating from the SVC, LAA or CS, in which cases complete isolation of these structures is the ablation strategy of choice.

Left Atrial Posterior Wall

The left atrial PW is that area of the left atrium located between the right and left PVs. From an embryologic, anatomic, and electrophysiological standpoint, it should be considered an extension of the PVs.[5] Therefore, empirical isolation of the left atrial PW should be performed in all patients undergoing first-time AF ablation, including patients with paroxysmal AF. For patients with nonparoxysmal AF or those undergoing repeat ablation with an isolated PW, its isolation is usually extended more anteriorly, to the mid-anterior wall and mid-septal areas, and inferiorly, to floor of the left atrium down to the endocardial aspect of the CS (**Fig. 2**). The endpoint is to achieve electrical isolation, as documented by the absence of any electrical activity in the PW and neighboring targeted areas.

Of note, the PW is in close relationship with the esophagus: to reduce the risk of esophageal damage and atrioesophageal fistula, it is important to know its location during the procedure (with intracardiac echocardiography [ICE] or contrast esophagography), use real-time temperature monitoring, and titrate power and/or contact force while moving the catheter quickly along the entire PW. It is also important to remember that the esophagus is wider than the temperature probe, therefore sometimes no or minimal temperature change is recorded, despite ablating over the esophagus; thus, it is good practice to move quickly whenever ablating the posterior/inferior

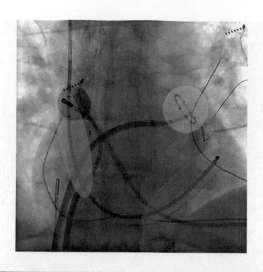

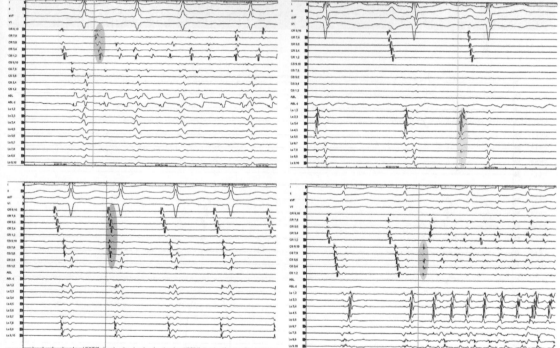

Fig. 1. Mapping of non-PV triggers. *Top,* fluoroscopy showing the catheter position during high-dose isoproterenol infusion; bottom, PAC from the SVC triggering AF (*green*); PAC from the IAS (*magenta*); PAC from the LAA (*yellow*); PAC from the CS triggering AF (*blue*). (*Adapted from* Gianni C, Mohanty S, Trivedi C, Di Biase L, Natale A. Novel concepts and approaches in ablation of atrial fibrillation: the role of non-pulmonary vein triggers. *EP Eur.* 2018;20(10):1566-1576; with permission.)

LA (including the CS), regardless of the location of the esophageal probe.

Superior Vena Cava

A common site of non-PV triggers is the SVC. Empirical SVC isolation is a reasonable addition to PVAI even in patients with paroxysmal AF and should be performed in every patient demonstrating firing originating from the SVC. As for the PVs, SVC isolation is preferred to focal ablation, which is time consuming, not as effective, and carries the risk of SVC stenosis with secondary SVC syndrome. To perform SVC isolation (**Fig. 3**), the CMC is positioned at the junction between the right atrium and SVC, with potentials

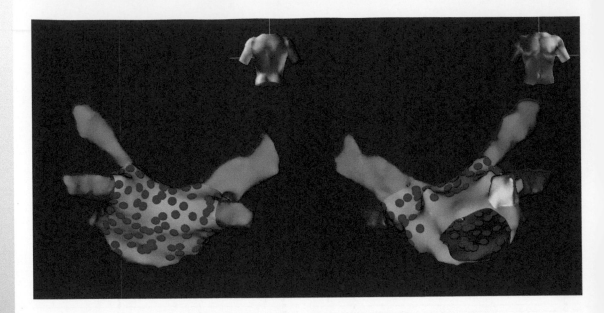

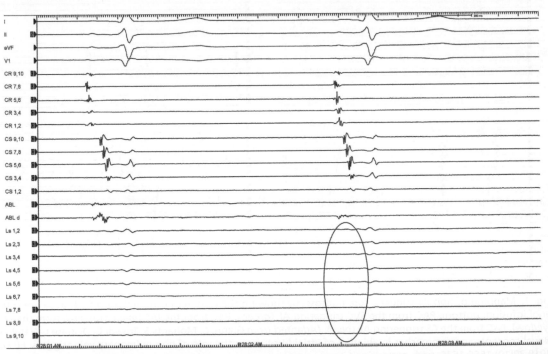

Fig. 2. Left atrial PW isolation at the time of repeat PVAI. *Top*, lesion set for left atrial PW isolation, which is extended inferiorly down to the CS, and anteriorly, to the mid-IAS and anterior wall. *Bottom*, intracardiac electrograms of the CMC (Ls) positioned in the PW after its electrical isolation. (*Adapted from* Gianni C, Mohanty S, Trivedi C, Di Biase L, Natale A. Novel concepts and approaches in ablation of atrial fibrillation: the role of non-pulmonary vein triggers. *EP Eur.* 2018;20(10):1566-1576; with permission.)

resembling that of the PVs, with a sharp vein potential superimposed to a blunt far-field atrial electrogram. ICE can help define the SVC-right atrial junction by visualizing the CMC between the right superior PV and the right pulmonary artery. SVC

isolation can be achieved with a segmental approach starting on the septal aspect. When targeting the lateral aspect, phrenic nerve mapping with high-output bipolar pacing is performed beforehand (of note, under general anesthesia

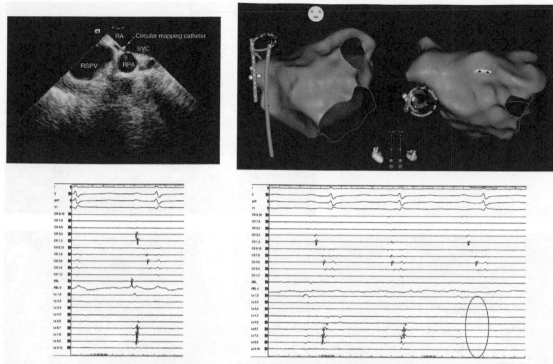

Fig. 3. Ablation of the SVC. *Top left*, ICE showing the CMC positioned at the junction between the SVC and RA; *top right*, lesion set for SVC isolation, which was achieved targeting the septal aspect of the SVC-RA junction (*white dots*, phrenic nerve mapping); *bottom*, intracardiac electrograms of the CMC (Ls) positioned in the SVC, at baseline (*left*) and showing (*right*) its delay (first and second beat) and isolation (third beat on). (*Adapted from* Gianni C, Mohanty S, Trivedi C, Di Biase L, Natale A. Novel concepts and approaches in ablation of atrial fibrillation: the role of non-pulmonary vein triggers. *EP Eur.* 2018;20(10):1566-1576; with permission.)

paralytic agents should be avoided or pacing performed after an adequate wash-out), and ff the phrenic nerve is captured on the lateral aspect of the SVC, another approach targeting the right atrial posterior wall can be used.[6] Another possible complication is damage of the sinus node, which lies laterally below the SVC: if acceleration of the sinus rate is observed during ablation (a sign of impending sinus node injury), radiofrequency (RF) energy should be discontinued. As for the PVs, endpoint is complete isolation with documented entrance conduction block.

Special mention merits to the subset of patients with left persistent SVC (LPSVC). Its isolation should be considered as first-line treatment in all patients, given its arrhythmogenicity and close relation with other important left atrial structures (left PVs and LAA).[7,8] Isolation of the LPSVC is guided by the CMC that can be easily advanced through a dilated CS reaching the level of the left superior PV/LAA ridge (**Fig. 4**). The CMC is continuously pulled back while performing electrogram-guided ablation: LPSVC isolation is usually performed along with CS isolation (see later

discussion), with the endpoint of obtaining dissociation or abolition of sharp potentials along the 2 structures. In these patients, the CS is dilated, and the CMC might not be in good contact with the entire vessel wall for any given position: for this reason, it is important to manipulate the catheter around the wall to confirm the absence of sharp vein potentials. Moreover, careful left phrenic nerve mapping as well as monitoring the esophageal temperature should always be performed, as the dilated CS and LPSVC are in close relationship with both structures.

Coronary Sinus

Non-PV triggers originating from the CS are common in patients with persistent AF and long-standing persistent AF, and its empirical isolation should be considered as a first-line therapy and performed at the time of repeat ablation. CS isolation is challenging, given the presence of myocardial sleeves that surround it connecting the CS to the left atrium.[9] Therefore, to achieve complete CS isolation it is important to target the vessel

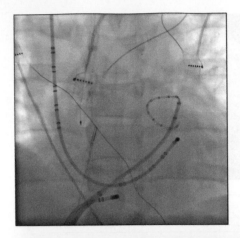
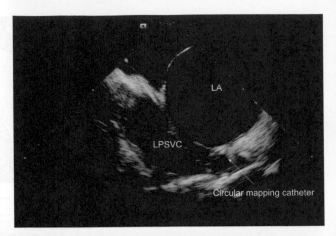
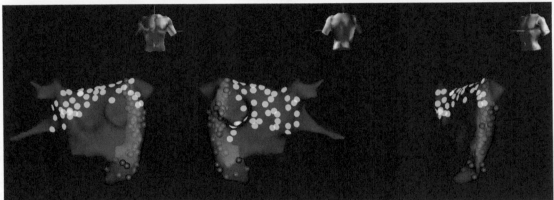

Fig. 4. Ablation of the LPSVC. *Top*, fluoroscopy and ICE images of the CMC positioned within the LPSVC; *bottom*, lesion set for LPSVC/CS isolation in a patient with PAF. (*Adapted from* Gianni C, Mohanty S, Trivedi C, Di Biase L, Natale A. Novel concepts and approaches in ablation of atrial fibrillation: the role of non-pulmonary vein triggers. *EP Eur.* 2018;20(10):1566-1576; with permission.)

both endocardially and epicardially (**Fig. 5**). Endocardial ablation is performed in the anterior aspect of the inferolateral LA, with the ablation catheter positioned at the level of the mitral valve annulus, parallel to the one positioned in the CS. Ablation is performed with the endpoint of elimination of local sharp electrograms spanning from the lateral left atrium to the septum, adjacent to the CS os (this usually requires looping the catheter up to 180°). Epicardial ablation, inside the CS, is started distally, and the ablation catheter is continuously dragged back to the CS os, making sure the catheter tip is freely moving, and not wedged in a small branch to avoid steam pops (any sudden impedance increase from the baseline should prompt RF discontinuation). The procedural endpoint is complete isolation, as demonstrated by dissociation or abolition of any potentials along the CS body.

Of note, an important precaution should be taken when ablating proximally in the CS, given the vicinity of the AV node: beat-to-beat PR monitoring is crucial, with immediate RF energy discontinuation in case of PR prolongation. The CS is also in close relationship with the esophagus, thus real-time esophageal temperature monitoring should be performed to avoid the possible formation of cardioesophageal fistulas.[10]

Left Atrial Appendage

Non-PV triggers can originate from the LAA, with their prevalence increasing in patients with nonparoxysmal AF: indeed, empirical LAA isolation can be considered as a first-line approach for patients with long-standing persistent AF.[11] Again, given the high recurrence rates in patients undergoing focal ablation, LAA isolation is to be preferred.

LAA isolation can be achieved with a technique similar to that of PVI, although it is more challenging given the wide variability of the LAA ostial anatomy. The CMC is positioned at the level of the LAA ostium (as easily assessed by ICE), and

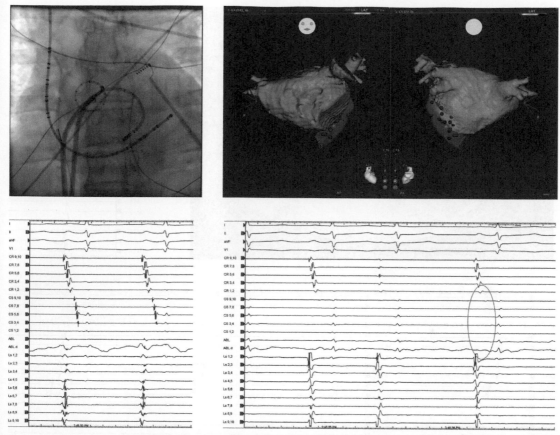

Fig. 5. Ablation of the CS. *Top left,* fluoroscopy image of the ablation catheter position to effectively target the CS endocardially; *top right,* lesion set for epicardial CS ablation; *bottom,* intracardiac electrograms showing the CS before (*left*) and after (*right*) its isolation (of note, with a PAC originating from the LAA). (*Adapted from Gianni C, Mohanty S, Trivedi C, Di Biase L, Natale A. Novel concepts and approaches in ablation of atrial fibrillation: the role of non-pulmonary vein triggers. EP Eur. 2018;20(10):1566-1576; with permission.*)

ablation is performed targeting the earliest LAA activation site, aiming for delay until complete isolation with entrance block is documented (**Fig. 6**). This is preferably done during sinus rhythm, when it is easier to define the LA-LAA breakthrough. A contact force sensing ablation catheter is helpful to ensure adequate catheter tip-tissue contact. It is also important not to advance the CMC deep into the LAA to avoid ablation inside the LAA: the wall is thin between the pectinate muscles, and the risk of perforation and left phrenic nerve injury is heightened.

With persistent LAA isolation, its mechanical function is impaired despite maintenance of sinus rhythm; therefore, patients should continue long-term oral anticoagulation or be considered for LAA occlusion.

Other Sites

Other common locations of non-PV triggers are the CR, IAS, ligament of Marshall (LoM), and mitral and tricuspid valve annuli, but foci can originate anywhere in the atria, especially in patients with atriopathy.[12,13] These triggers are usually targeted with focal ablation after activation mapping identifies the site of origin, the endpoint being termination/noninducibility of the AT or disappearance of the repetitive PACs. Exception is for triggers originating from LoM, where isolation along the whole ligament is the endpoint of choice. The LoM is an epicardial vestigial fold that marks the location of the embryologic left SVC and contains the vein of Marshall, nerves, and muscular fibers.[14] It runs from the mid-distal CS through the posterolateral LA, up to the epicardial aspect of the ridge between the left superior PV and LAA. It is possible to target the LoM area endocardially by ablation in the mid-lateral LA (between the CS and left inferior PV) up to the ridge.[15] Alternatively, direct ethanol injection in the vein of Marshall has shown to be an effective way to achieve ablation along the whole LoM without significant complications.[16]

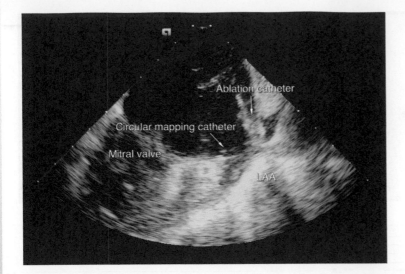
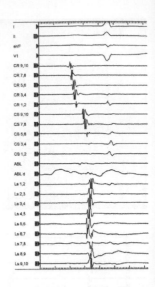
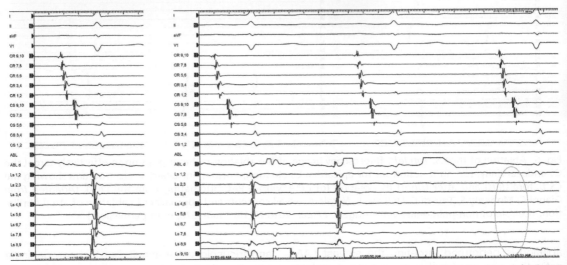

Fig. 6. Ablation of the LAA. *Top left*, ICE showing the CMC positioned at the ostium of the LAA; *top right*, intracardiac electrograms of the CMC (Ls) at baseline; *bottom*, intracardiac electrograms of the CMC (Ls) showing LAA delay (*left*) and isolation (*right*). (*Adapted from* Gianni C, Mohanty S, Trivedi C, Di Biase L, Natale A. Novel concepts and approaches in ablation of atrial fibrillation: the role of non-pulmonary vein triggers. *EP Eur.* 2018;20(10):1566-1576; with permission.)

SUMMARY

Ablation of non-PV triggers is an important step to improve outcomes in AF ablation. Non-PV triggers typically originate from predictable sites (such as the left atrial PW, SVC, CS, IAS, CR), and these areas can be ablated either empirically or after observing significant ectopy (with or without drug challenge). Mapping of non-PV triggers can be performed quickly with the aid of multielectrode catheters positioned in key areas of the right atrium and left atrium. They can be targeted with focal ablation, exception being the triggers originating from the SVC, LAA, or CS, for which complete isolation is the ablation strategy of choice.

DISCLOSURE

No relevant conflicts of interest to disclose.

REFERENCES

1. Haegeli LM, Calkins H. Catheter ablation of atrial fibrillation: an update. EurHeart J 2014;35(36): 2454–9.

2. Gianni C, Mohanty S, Trivedi C, et al. Novel con-cepts and approaches in ablation of atrial fibrillation: the role of non-pulmonary vein triggers. Europace 2018;20(10):1566–76.

3. Blom NA, Gittenberger-de Groot AC, DeRuiter MC, et al. Development of the cardiac conduction tissue in human embryos using HNK-1 antigen expression: possible relevance for understanding of abnormal atrial automaticity. Circulation 1999;99(6):800–6.

4. De Simone CV, Noheria A, Lachman N, et al. Myocardium of the superior vena cava, coronary si-nus, vein of marshall, and the pulmonary vein ostia: gross anatomic studies in 620 hearts. J CardiovascElectrophysiol 2012;23(12):1304–9.

5. Urena M, Rodés-Cabau J, Freixa X, et al. Percuta-neous left atrial appendage closure with the AM-PLATZER cardiac plug device in patients with nonvalvular atrial fibrillation and contraindications to anticoagulation therapy. J Am CollCardiol 2013; 62(2):96–102.

6. Gianni C, Sanchez JE, Mohanty S, et al. Isolation of the superior vena cava from the right atrial posterior wall: a novel ablation approach. Europace 2018; 20(9):e124–32.

7. Hsu L-F. Atrial fibrillation originating from persistent left superior vena cava. Circulation 2004;109(7): 828–32.

8. Elayi CS, Fahmy TS, Wazni OM, et al. Left superior vena cava isolation in patients undergoing pulmo-nary vein antrum isolation: impact on atrial fibrillation recurrence. Heart Rhythm 2006;3(9):1019–23.

9. Ho SY, Sánchez-Quintana D, Becker AE. A review of the coronary venous system: a road less travelled. Heart Rhythm 2004;1(1):107–12.

10. Güneş MF, Gökoğlan Y, Di Biase L, et al. Ablating the posterior heart: cardioesophageal fistula compli-cating radiofrequency ablation in the coronary sinus. J CardiovascElectrophysiol 2015;26(12):1376–8.

11. Di Biase L, Burkhardt JD, Mohanty P, et al. Left atrial appendage isolation in patients with longstanding persistent AF undergoing catheter ablation: BELIEF trial. J Am CollCardiol 2016;68(18):1929–40.

12. Lin WS, Tai CT, Hsieh MH, et al. Catheter ablation of paroxysmal atrial fibrillation initiated by non-pulmonary vein ectopy. Circulation 2003;107(25): 3176–83.

13. Lee SH, Chen SA, Tai CT. Predictors of non-pulmonary vein ectopic beats initiating paroxysmal atrial fibrillation - Implication for catheter ablation. ActaCardiolSin 2007;23(1):13–9.

14. Kim DT, Lai AC, Hwang C, et al. The ligament of Marshall: a structural analysis in human hearts with implications for atrial arrhythmias. J Am CollCardiol 2000;36(4):1324–7.

15. Kurotobi T, Ito H, Inoue K, et al. Marshall vein as ar-rhythmogenic source in patients with atrial fibrillation: correlation between its anatomy and electrophysio-logical findings. J CardiovascElectrophysiol 2006; 17(10):1062–7.

16. Dave AS, Báez-Escudero JL, Sasaridis C, et al. Role of the vein of Marshall in atrial fibrillation recurrences after catheter ablation: therapeutic effect of ethanol infusion. J CardiovascElectrophysiol 2012;23(6): 583–91.

Beyond Pulmonary Vein Isolation in Nonparoxysmal Atrial Fibrillation

Posterior Wall, Vein of Marshall, Coronary Sinus, Superior Vena Cava, and Left Atrial Appendage

David F. Briceño, MD[a], Kavisha Patel, MD[a], Jorge Romero, MD[a],
Isabella Alviz, MD[a], Nicola Tarantino, MD[a], Domenico G. Della Rocca, MD[b],
Veronica Natale, BS[b], Xiao-Dong Zhang, MD[a],
Luigi Di Biase, MD, PhD, FHRS[a,*]

KEYWORDS

- Nonparoxysmal AF • Ablation • Posterior wall • LAA • Coronary sinus • SVC • Ligament of Marshall

KEY POINTS

- Pulmonary vein isolation (PVI) is the cornerstone of AF ablation but additional ablation is necessary in selected patients particularly in nonparoxysmal AF.
- Incidence of non-PV triggers is higher in female gender, older age, patients with obesity, obstructive sleep apnea, low left ventricular ejection fraction, severe left atrial scarring, hypertrophic cardiomyopathy, and mechanical mitral valve.
- Non-PV trigger sites include superior vena cava, posterior wall, left atrial appendage, coronary sinus, vein of Marshall, crista terminalis/Eustachian ridge, interatrial septum, and mitral and tricuspid annuli.
- Non-PV trigger sites are targeted empirically in selected cases or if significant ectopy is noted (with or without a drug challenge).
- Elimination of non-PV triggers by means of focal ablation at the site of origin or isolation of arrhythmogenic structures has been associated with improved arrhythmia-free survival.
- The PLEA trial, a prospective, randomized, multicenter trial (ClinicalTrials.gov identifier: NCT04216667), which is the largest trial assessing most of these ablation strategies for nonparoxysmal AF, will clarify the role of these approaches.

INTRODUCTION

Atrial fibrillation (AF) is the most common cardiac rhythm disturbance,[1] which is estimated to affect approximately 33 million individuals worldwide.[2] By 2050, estimates have projected that the prevalence of AF in the United States alone would increase to 5.6 to 15.9 million individuals.[3,4] Mortality rates among patients with AF remain up to two-fold higher than individuals without AF.[5,6] AF also has a detrimental effect on quality of

[a] Montefiore Medical Center, Albert Einstein College of Medicine, 111 East 210th Street, Bronx, NY 10467, USA; [b] Texas Cardiac Arrhythmia Institute, St. David's Medical Center, Austin, TX, USA
* Corresponding author.
E-mail address: dibbia@gmail.com

Card Electrophysiol Clin 12 (2020) 219–231
https://doi.org/10.1016/j.ccep.2020.01.002

life, with a well-recognized increased risk of thromboembolic events[7] and heart failure. The 2017 HRS/EHRA/ECAS/APHRS/SOLAECE expert consensus statement on catheter and surgical ablation of AF recommend catheter ablation (CA) as the selected rhythm strategy in selected patients. In particular, CA is recommended for symptomatic persistent and long-standing persistent (LSP) AF (LSPAF) either as an initial strategy or refractory or intolerant to at least one class I or III antiarrhythmic medications (class IIa and IIb recommendations, respectively).[8] In the setting of heart failure with reduced ejection fraction, multiple studies have already shown major benefit in all-cause mortality of CA.[9] The studies assessing the benefit of CA in persistent AF[10–13] and LSPAF[14,15] have been limited by a substantial degree of heterogeneity given varying sample sizes, population subgroups, and outcomes assessed. Considerable variation has been observed in short- and long-term success rates using different techniques, and the most optimal strategy to be pursued still remains to be determined.

Two decades ago, a landmark study[16] established that the pulmonary veins (PVs) are the most frequent trigger source of AF, which was the emergence of PV isolation (PVI) as the cornerstone of CA for AF. This strategy eventually developed into an antral approach to minimize complications (PVAI). Although PVAI alone may be enough in patients with paroxysmal AF (where PVs are frequently the only trigger source), it has been suggested that this is not sufficient to treat patients with nonparoxysmal AF.[17] In a recent prospective study[18] of approximately 2100 patients, AF initiation from non-PV trigger sources was demonstrated in approximately 11% of patients with persistent and LSPAF referred for CA. The concept that AF recurrences can occur in patients with isolated PVs on repeat procedures, from non-PV trigger sites, was also corroborated by another study of approximately 500 patients with AF followed over a decade.[19] Non-PV trigger sources have been identified to arise from different sites. Herein, the evidence and ablation strategies for non-PV triggers from the following sites are reviewed: the posterior wall (PW) of the left atrium (LA), the left atrial appendage (LAA), the coronary sinus (CS), the superior vena cava (SVC), and the left SVC and its remnant-vein of Marshall (VOM) (**Fig. 1**).[18,19]

IDENTIFICATION OF NONPULMONARY VEIN TRIGGERS

Non-PV triggers are sites that typically contain myocardial cells with arrhythmogenic properties.[20,21] This is caused by a combination of enhanced automaticity,[20] triggered activity,[22] and microreentrant circuits.[23] A higher prevalence of non-PV triggers has been noted in patients with nonparoxysmal AF, female gender, older age, patients with obesity, obstructive sleep apnea, low left ventricular ejection fraction, severe left atrial scarring, hypertrophic cardiomyopathy, and mechanical mitral valve.[24] In this subset of patients, it is recommended that non-PV triggers be targeted at the time of the index procedure.[25–34]

Discontinuation of anti-arrhythmic drugs five half-lives before the procedure is recommended to prevent noninducibility of these triggers. Given the transient nature of non-PV triggers and its quick degeneration to AF, detailed activation map creation using multiple mapping catheters is crucial (**Fig. 2**). Localization of non-PV foci involves a detailed analysis of specific intra-atrial activation sequences using multipolar catheters in standard atrial locations coupled with information from the surface electrocardiogram P wave when possible. Multipolar catheters positioned along the CS and crista terminalis/SVC region together with direct recordings from the right and left PVs allow a quick localization of non-PV foci.

Prior studies have reported a variable degree of prevalence of non-PV trigger sites, governed by the rigorousness of the stimulation protocol adopted and the definition adopted for a significant trigger (only ectopic beats that can reliably initiate AF vs frequent ectopic beats without initiating AF). It has been argued that a protocol using high doses of isoproterenol (20–30 μg/min) is necessary to induce consistent non-PV triggers. It has been well established to target non-PV triggers that lead to sustained AF/atrial flutter (AFL) or cause reproducible initiation of nonsustained AF.[35] Additionally, improved outcomes have been reported by some centers also targeting repeated isolated premature atrial contractions and nonsustained focal atrial tachycardias (ATs).[35]

POSTERIOR WALL

The PW of the LA is considered an embryologic sibling of the PVs.[36] In patients with AF, the PW undergoes progressive remodeling over time. This concept is substantiated by microscopic evidence, with a greater extent of lymphonuclear/fatty infiltration, and fibrosis noted in patients with persistent AF.[37–39] Cellular evidence includes presence of increased occurrence of delayed depolarizations, increased late sodium, and calcium currents resulting in larger calcium content of sarcoplasmic reticulum.[40] This substrate eventually leads to greater spontaneous triggered activity, and propulsion of fibrillatory impulses to both

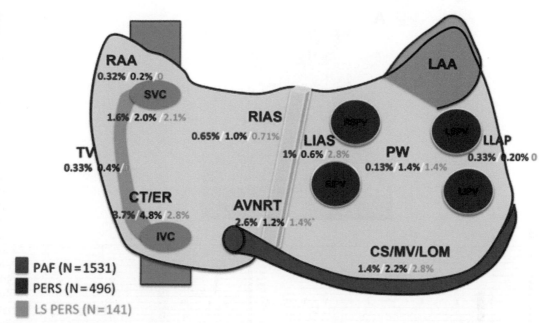

Fig. 1. Prevalence of sustained and nonsustained triggers from nonpulmonary veins according to different atrial fibrillation types. AVNRT, AV node re-entrant tachycardia; CT, crista terminalis; ER, eustacian ridge; LIAS, left interatrial septum; LIPV, left inferior pulmonary vein; LLAP, left lateral accessory pathway; LOM, ligament of Marshall; LS PERS, long-standing persistent; LSPV, left superior pulmonary vein; MV, mitral valve; PAF, paroxysmal atrial fibrillation; PERS, persistent; RAA, right atrial appendage; RIAS, right interatrial septum; RIPV, right inferior pulmonary vein; RSPV, right superior pulmonary vein; TV, tricuspid valve. [a] Two patients with longstanding persistent AF. (*From* Santangeli P, Zado ES, Hutchinson MD, Riley MP, Lin D, Frankel DS, Supple GE, Garcia FC, Dixit S, Callans DJ, Marchlinski FE. Prevalence and distribution of focal triggers in persistent and long-standing persistent atrial fibrillation. Heart Rhythm 2016;13:374–382; with permission.)

atria. Despite the growing evidence that effective PW isolation would lead to better outcomes in patients with persistent AF,[41–45] this strategy has not been widely adopted. Proven isolation of the PW provides additional benefits over PVAI alone in the treatment of persistent AF and improves procedural outcome at follow-up. However, this strategy is still associated with a significant high incidence of very late recurrence of atrial tachyarrhythmia, suggesting the need for more extensive ablation, perhaps trigger based, in selected patients.[41] A recent meta-analysis of seven studies with a total of 1151 patients was recently published showing the benefits of PW isolation. In this study, patients who underwent concomitant PW isolation experienced less recurrence of all-atrial arrhythmias postablation (relative risk [RR], 0.77; 95% confidence interval [CI], 0.62–0.96; *P* = .02) and less recurrence of AF (RR, 0.55; 95% CI, 0.39–0.77; *P* < .01). There was no difference in onset of AT/AFL (RR, 0.96; 95% CI, 0.62–1.48; *P* = .85) after ablation. These results were replicated in subgroup analysis of patients with persistent AF.[46]

The optimal strategy to accomplish PW isolation has been debated. Linear ablation (box lesion set with roof and inferior lines) has been a suggested strategy but it is technically difficult; even a single gap can lead to reconnection of the entire PW with the rest of the LA.[47] In addition, it is not unusual to encounter epicardial connections in the middle of the PW between both lines. As such, electrogram-based ablation has been reported where all signals identified on the mapping catheter are sequentially targeted (**Fig. 3**). End point is to achieve electrical isolation of the PW with bidirectional block (see **Fig. 3**). Given the close relationship between the esophagus and the PW of the LA, continuous esophageal temperature monitoring is imperative. Because the esophagus is wider than the temperature probe, it is also recommended to move the ablation catheter promptly while creating lesions on the PW, because no or minimal temperature change may be seen despite delivering RF energy directly over the esophagus. Concern for deterioration of LA contractile function has been raised with extensive PW ablation. However, LA contractility is - primarily a function of the muscular anterior, septal inferior, and lateral walls with negligible contribution from the PW. As such, no decline in LA function has been reported after extensive

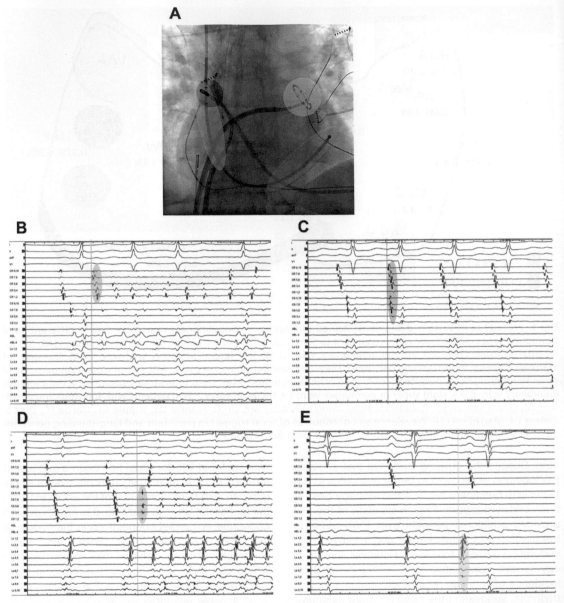

Fig. 2. Mapping of non-PV triggers. (*A*) Catheter position during high-dose isoproterenol infusion. (*B*) PAC from the SVC triggering AF. (*C*) PAC from the interatrial septum. (*D*) PAC from the CS triggering AF. (*E*) PAC from the LAA. *Green,* SVC/crista terminalis; *magenta,* interatrial septum; *blue,* CS; *yellow,* LAA. PAC, premature atrial contraction. (*From* Gianni, C, Mohanty S, Trivedi C, Di Biase L, Natale A. Novel concepts and approaches in ablation of atrial fibrillation: the role of non-pulmonary vein triggers. Europace, 2018. 20(10): p. 1566-1576; with permission.)

PW ablation.[48] Cryoablation of PW also seems to be a safe, effective, and feasible alternative strategy to RF energy. In a prospective, nonrandomized study of 390 patients, second-generation cryoballoon ablation showed higher rate of freedom from atrial arrhythmias for patients undergoing PW + PVI, compared with patients that underwent PVI alone (hazard ratio, 2.04; 95% CI, 1.15–3.61; P = .015); complication rates were similar between the two groups.[49] PIVoTAL, a prospective, randomized, multicenter trial (ClinicalTrials.gov identifier: NCT03057548), is presently under way to evaluate the incremental benefit of cryoablation of PW isolation in addition to PVI. Considering inconsistent results even from randomized trials assessing the role of PW ablation, further trials are eagerly awaited. The PLEA trial, a prospective, randomized, multicenter trial (ClinicalTrials.gov identifier: NCT04216667), which is the largest trial assessing different

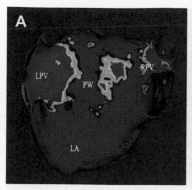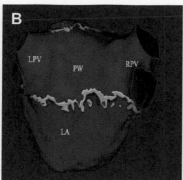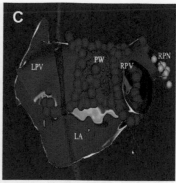

Fig. 3. Ablation of PW of the LA. (*A*) Preablation voltage map with scar tissue in the posterior wall. (*B*) Postablation voltage map following PVI and PW isolation. (*C*) Lesion set for PW and PVI ablation. Note that for PW isolation, additional electrograms were targeted after creating inferior and roof lines. LPV, left pulmonary veins; RPN, right phrenic nerve; RPV, right pulmonary veins.

ablation strategies for nonparoxysmal AF, will explore this ablation approach.

SUPERIOR VENA CAVA

SVC is an important site of initiation of non-PV triggers.[50,51] Embryologically, it originates from right sinus horn (origin of sinoatrial node); therefore, SVC tissue is capable of spontaneous firing.[52] SVC isolation has been shown to improve outcomes when added to PVAI in patients with either documented SVC triggers or as an empirical strategy in paroxysmal and nonparoxysmal AF.[50,53,54]

A prospective, randomized study of 320 patients with paroxysmal and nonparoxysmal AF[54] evaluated the role of empirical SVC isolation in addition to PVAI during index ablation; at 12-month follow-up, the procedural success rate was better solely in patients with paroxysmal AF (77% vs 90%; $P = .04$). Furthermore, in a nonrandomized study[55] of 70 patients with persistent AF, PVI alone was sufficient to suppress AF in only approximately 56% patients, at a median follow-up of approximately 32 months. During second and third repeat procedures, higher success was achieved with SVC isolation (in cases with no PV reconnection) than with only repeat PV reisolation (74% vs 66%). Because AF is a progressive disease, with increasing electrical and structural remodeling from paroxysmal to persistent to LSPAF, targeting SVC triggers in addition to PVAI is not enough in nonparoxysmal AF.[56,57]

To improve effectiveness, procedural time, and decrease risk of SVC stenosis/SVC syndrome, SVC circumferential isolation is recommended as opposed to multifocal ablation of triggers originating from muscular sleeves. While performing SVC isolation, the mapping catheter is positioned at the SVC/right atrium (RA) junction. Intracardiac

echocardiography can offer enhanced anatomic orientation for this purpose. Ectopic beats originating from SVC demonstrate earliest activation at the proximal bipole of duodecapolar catheter with a clear proximal-to-distal (SVC-RA/crista terminalis (CT)-CS) sequence. Conversely, triggers originating from upper CT or right superior PV show early activation at distal poles of the duodecapolar catheter located adjacent to RA/CT.

SVC isolation is achieved using a segmental approach, using radiofrequency (RF) energy, commencing on the septal aspect (**Fig. 4**). While ablating the lateral aspect, it is crucial to avoid injury to the phrenic nerve and the sinus node. Phrenic nerve mapping is performed at high output pacing ($\geq$20 mA); it is important to avoid paralytic agents under general anesthesia or pacing should be performed after a sufficient washout period (see **Fig. 4**). In up to 10% of patients, complete isolation of SVC is not possible because of risk of phrenic nerve injury. In such patients, ablation of right atrial PW is used alternatively.[58] The sinus node lies laterally below the SVC; RF energy delivery should promptly be discontinued if acceleration of the sinus rate is noted (an imminent sign of sinus node injury). It is also imperative to not perform ablation during isoproterenol infusion to avoid masking injury to sinus node. End point of SVC ablation is complete isolation (see **Fig. 4**) with documented entrance/exit block.

CORONARY SINUS

In patients with persistent AF and LSPAF, some evidence suggests that the CS is a frequent trigger source for AF.[59–62] Myocardial connections of varying numbers and morphology have been demonstrated between the CS and the LA on necropsied hearts.[63] The distal aspect of the muscular sleeve

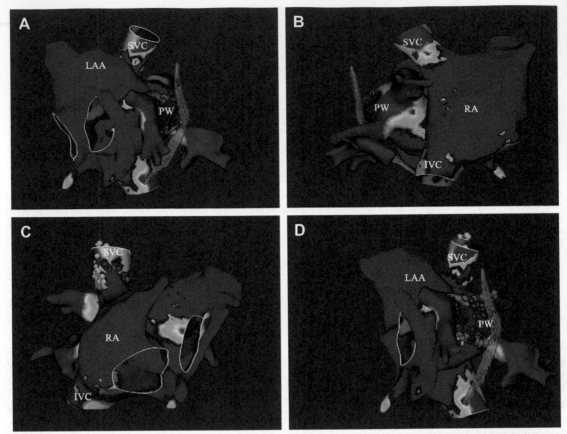

Fig. 4. Ablation of SVC. (*A, B*) Postablation voltage map following PVI, SVC, and PW isolation. (*A*) Left lateral view. (*B*) Right lateral view. (*C, D*) Lesion set for PW, PVI ,and SVC ablation. Note the circumferential lesion set (*blue dots*) and the details of phrenic nerve mapping (*yellow dots*) using high output pacing. IVC, inferior vena cava; RA, right atrium.

for the CS usually terminates at valve of Vieussens, covering the drainage site for the posterolateral vein and is the anatomic landmark between the CS and the great cardiac vein.[64] This muscular sleeve can potentially serve as an ectopic trigger or may form part of a reentrant circuit for AF.[65] The concept that electrical disconnection of the CS from the LA would lower the inducibility of AF was first substantiated more than a decade ago.[59] Patients with higher frequency signal in the proximal CS and a lower distal CS/proximal CS frequency ratio (with a cutoff of 67%) were recently noted to have a higher likelihood of AF-free survival after CS ablation.[66] This study performed CS ablation only using the endocardial approach.

Some authors advocate to target the vessel endocardially and epicardially. Given the variable anatomy and therefore, varying CS trigger sites for AF, focal ablation is more challenging and time-consuming. In a study of 225 patients undergoing PVI for AF, at approximately 21 months of follow-up, complete isolation of CS demonstrated a higher freedom from AF than focal

ablation of triggers (74% vs 51%; *P*<0.001). Despite a higher fluoroscopic time, RF energy delivery time and total procedural time with complete isolation, it is a more desirable approach given similar safety and a much higher efficacy profile. Despite these results, data from randomized clinical trials are still lacking. The PLEA trial, a prospective, randomized, multicenter trial (ClinicalTrials.gov identifier: NCT04216667), which is the largest trial assessing different ablation strategies for nonparoxysmal AF, will explore this ablation approach.

Endocardial ablation is performed starting from the anterior portion of inferolateral aspect of LA close to the mitral annulus; parallel to the CS. The ablation catheter is dragged from the lateral to the septal aspect (may necessitate 180° looping of the catheter) with the aim to abolish sharp electrograms along the CS (**Fig. 5**). While performing epicardial ablation from within the CS, the catheter tip should be directed posteriorly where the muscular connections from the CS to LA are present. It is important to avoid directing it anteriorly because there is risk of injury to the coronary artery. Epicardial ablation is started at the distal end of the CS and the catheter is dragged along the length of the vessel up to the ostium (see **Fig. 5**). It is crucial to ensure that the tip of the catheter moves freely and does not get lodged in a small vessel to prevent steam pops. Any increase in impedance should lead to immediate discontinuation of RF delivery. End point is achieved when there is complete abolishment or dissociation of signals along the body of CS. Given the close relationship between the esophagus and the CS, continuous esophageal temperature monitoring is important to avoid complications.[67] While ablating along the septal aspect, close monitoring of PR interval is pertinent with prompt RF energy discontinuation with any signs of PR prolongation to avoid injury to the atrioventricular nodal artery.

LEFT ATRIAL APPENDAGE

About a decade ago, the LAA was first identified as an underrecognized trigger site of AF.[68,69] In a study of 987 patients undergoing redo AF ablation, 27% patients were noted to have firing from the LAA; in 8.7% of cases, it was the only source of atrial arrhythmia with no PV or extra-PV reconnection.[68] The BELIEF trial,[70] a randomized study designed to assess the benefit of empiric LAA electrical isolation (LAAEI) in patients with LSPAF, reported improved freedom from atrial arrhythmias in single and redo procedures. Incremental benefit of LAAEI in addition to PVI was also demonstrated in two meta-analyses[71,72] involving approximately 2000 patients with persistent AF and LSPAF. Complete LAAEI was associated with a lower arrhythmia recurrence compared with focal ablation (15% vs 68% at 12-month follow-up),[68]

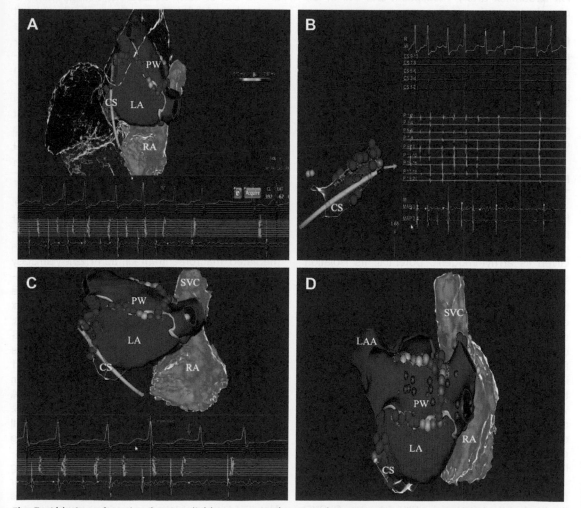

Fig. 5. Ablation of CS. (*A–C*) Epicardial lesion set in the CS with termination of the arrhythmia (*red arrow*). (*D*) Postablation voltage map with the ablation lesion set in the PW and the CS. RA, right atrium.

without increasing the rates of complications. Some groups have raised thromboembolic complications as the major limitation of this approach.[73,74] Nonetheless, the safety of this approach has been consistently confirmed as long as appropriate anticoagulation is maintained or LAA occlusion is performed.[75]

To obtain LAAEI, the mapping catheter is positioned at the level of the LAA ostium (confirmed on intracardiac echocardiography) (**Fig. 6**); RF energy is delivered ostially circumferentially until complete isolation is achieved (see **Fig. 6**). The target is to achieve entrance/exit block. It is crucial to prevent mapping and ablation deep into the LAA; because it is a thin structure, ablation inside is associated with a higher risk of perforation and left phrenic nerve injury. Cryoballoon-based isolation has also been noted to be an effective strategy for LAAEI to improve arrhythmia-free survival; however, it has been reported to cause 4% of left circumflex artery vasospasm and 1% of left phrenic nerve injury.[72,76]

LAAEI leads to impairment of its mechanical function. Therefore, it is vital to continue long-term anticoagulation following LAAEI, even in patients with sinus rhythm, unless LAA contractility is preserved on 6-month follow-up transesophageal echocardiography (evidenced by consistent A waves, Doppler emptying velocities of $\geq$0.4 m/s).[75] Alternatively, LAA occlusion is considered to decrease thromboembolic risk.

PERSISTENT LEFT SUPERIOR VENA CAVA AND THE VEIN OF MARSHALL

Persistent left SVC (PLSVC) occurs in patients with persistent left superior cardinal vein, which normally regresses to VOM in most individuals.[77] Given its arrhythmogenic potential, its isolation should be performed as first-line treatment.[78] A recent study in patients with AF referred to two tertiary hospitals described the arrhythmogenic role of PLSVC. Among 3967 patients, PLSVC was present in 36 patients (0.9%). Thirty-two patients underwent RFCA and electrophysiology study focusing on PLSVC: PLSVC was the trigger of AF in 48.4% of patients. Cumulatively, PLSVC was a trigger or driver of AF in 22 patients (68.8%). Whether to ablate PLSVC was determined by the results of electrophysiology study, and no significant difference in the late recurrence rate was observed between patients who did and did not have either trigger or driver from PLSVC.[79]

Ablation of PLSVC is guided by advancing the mapping catheter through a dilated CS close to the level of the left superior PV/LAA ridge. PLSVC ablation is performed along with CS isolation with the end point of achieving dissociation/elimination of sharp vein potentials as described previously for epicardial CS isolation. It is important to confirm that the absence of sharp vein potentials is caused by true elimination of triggers and not secondary to poor contact inside the dilated CS. Left phrenic nerve mapping and simultaneous esophageal temperature monitoring is crucial given the close relationship of these structures to PLSVC. Data on the use of cryotherapy for isolation of SVC[80] and PLSVC[81,82] have been limited to a few cases but it seems to be a feasible alternative.

The VOM is a vestigial fold that marks the site of the embryologic left SVC. The VOM has been particularly important in the setting of atrial tachycardias and AFL post-AF ablation.[83] In most cases, VOM triggers can reliably be detected by direct cannulation of the CS with a multipolar catheter. Origination of an ectopic trigger from VOM is indirectly suggested by early activation of mid-CS, or early endocardial activation in the posterolateral LA between the mid-CS and left inferior PV or in the ridge between LAA and the left superior PV. LOM area is targeted endocardially by ablating the muscular connection between posterolateral LA and CS: ridge between mid-CS/left inferior PV, and LAA/left superior PV.[84] Direct ethanol injection into VOM has also been described.[85] Ethanol infusion of the vein of VOM allows for specific ablation of the VOM, its intrinsic electrical activity, the neighboring myocardium and associated PV connections, the mitral isthmus, and the associated parasympathetic innervation.[86] Chugh and colleagues[87] reported 56 patients in whom LOM was considered to be a therapeutic target based on pacing data suggesting VOM-mediated LA PV connections or mapping data suggesting VOM-mediated macroreentrant or focal tachycardias. A total of 13 patients had VOM-mediated tachycardia (nine macroreentrant and four focal). RF targeting the VOM was successful in all but two patients. In 31 patients with perimitral atrial flutter, venography showed a suitable VOM in 23, and 16 of them received VOM ethanol, which led to perimitral conduction block (with or without added RF) in 15 (94%). The VOM Ethanol Infusion for Persistent Atrial Fibrillation trial, a prospective, randomized, multicenter trial (ClinicalTrials.gov identifier: NCT01898221) assessing the impact of this approach in reduction of AF/flutter, is under way (has completed enrollment).

SUMMARY

Non-PV trigger ablation is an important step toward improving outcomes of patients with

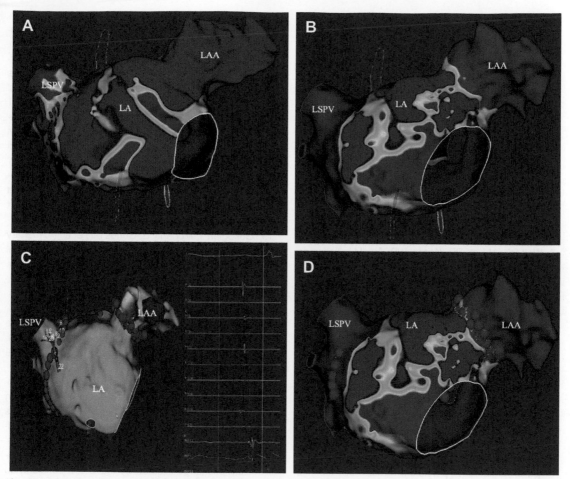

Fig. 6. LAA isolation. (*A*) Preablation map of the LA. (*B*) Postablation of the LA following PVI and LAA isolation. (*C*) Activation map showing the earliest point at the anterior wall of the LAA. (*D*) Postablation voltage map with the ablation lesion set in the PV and the LAA. LSPV, left superior pulmonary vein.

nonparoxysmal AF. Non-PV triggers typically originate from PW of the LA, SVC, LAA, VOM, CS, and other sites, such as the interatrial septum, crista terminalis/Eustachian ridge, and mitral and tricuspid valve annuli. These sites should be targeted when a trigger has been clearly identified, but empirical ablation is reasonable in selected cases. Most of these triggers are targeted with focal ablation. However, ablation of SVC, LAA, and CS should target complete isolation of these structures to improve atrial arrhythmia-free survival. A trial assessing the role of each of these strategies is eagerly awaited. The PLEA trial, a prospective, randomized, multicenter trial (ClinicalTrials.gov identifier: NCT04216667), which is the largest trial assessing most of these ablation strategies for nonparoxysmal AF, will clarify the role of these approaches.

DISCLOSURE

Dr L. Di Biase is a consultant for Stereotaxis, Biosense Webster, Boston Scientific, and Abbott Medical; and received speaker honoraria/travel support from Medtronic, Pfizer, Bristol Meyers Squibb, and Biotronik. The other authors have no disclosures.

REFERENCES

1. Wyndham CR. Atrial fibrillation: the most common arrhythmia. Tex Heart Inst J 2000;27(3):257–67.
2. Chugh SS, Havmoeller R, Narayanan K, et al. Worldwide epidemiology of atrial fibrillation: a global burden of disease 2010 study. Circulation 2014; 129(8):837–47.
3. Miyasaka Y, Barnes ME, Gersh BJ, et al. Secular trends in incidence of atrial fibrillation in Olmsted County, Minnesota, 1980 to 2000, and implications

on the projections for future prevalence. Circulation 2006;114(2):119–25.

4. Go AS, Barnes ME, Gersh BJ, et al. Prevalence of diagnosed atrial fibrillation in adults: national implications for rhythm management and stroke prevention: the AnTicoagulation and Risk Factors in Atrial Fibrillation (ATRIA) Study. JAMA 2001;285(18):2370–5.

5. Odutayo A, Wong CX, Hsiao AJ, et al. Atrial fibrillation and risks of cardiovascular disease, renal disease, and death: systematic review and meta-analysis. BMJ 2016;354:i4482.

6. Conen D, Chae CU, Glynn RJ, et al. Risk of death and cardiovascular events in initially healthy women with new-onset atrial fibrillation. JAMA 2011;305(20):2080–7.

7. Wolf PA, Abbott RD, Kannel WB. Atrial fibrillation as an independent risk factor for stroke: the Framingham Study. Stroke 1991;22(8):983–8.

8. Calkins H, Hindricks G, Cappato R, et al. 2017 HRS/EHRA/ECAS/APHRS/SOLAECE expert consensus statement on catheter and surgical ablation of atrial fibrillation. Heart Rhythm 2017;14(10):e275–444.

9. Briceno DF, Markman TM, Lupercio F, et al. Catheter ablation versus conventional treatment of atrial fibrillation in patients with heart failure with reduced ejection fraction: a systematic review and meta-analysis of randomized controlled trials. J Interv Card Electrophysiol 2018;53(1):19–29.

10. Parkash R, Tang AS, Sapp JL, Wells G, et al. Approach to the catheter ablation technique of paroxysmal and persistent atrial fibrillation: a meta-analysis of the randomized controlled trials. J Cardiovasc Electrophysiol 2011;22(7):729–38.

11. Oral H, Pappone C, Chugh A, et al. Circumferential pulmonary-vein ablation for chronic atrial fibrillation. N Engl J Med 2006;354(9):934–41.

12. Mont L, Bisbal F, Hernandez-Madrid A, et al. Catheter ablation vs. antiarrhythmic drug treatment of persistent atrial fibrillation: a multicentre, randomized, controlled trial (SARA study). Eur Heart J 2014;35(8):501–7.

13. Stabile G, Bertaglia E, Senatore G, et al. Catheter ablation treatment in patients with drug-refractory atrial fibrillation: a prospective, multi-centre, randomized, controlled study (Catheter Ablation for the Cure of Atrial Fibrillation Study). Eur Heart J 2006;27(2):216–21.

14. Haissaguerre M, Hocini M, Sanders P, et al. Catheter ablation of long-lasting persistent atrial fibrillation: clinical outcome and mechanisms of subsequent arrhythmias. J Cardiovasc Electrophysiol 2005;16(11):1138–47.

15. Calkins H, Reynolds MR, Spector P, et al. Treatment of atrial fibrillation with antiarrhythmic drugs or radiofrequency ablation: two systematic literature reviews and meta-analyses. Circ Arrhythm Electrophysiol 2009;2(4):349–61.

16. Haissaguerre M, Jais P, Shah DC, et al. Spontaneous initiation of atrial fibrillation by ectopic beats originating in the pulmonary veins. N Engl J Med 1998;339(10):659–66.

17. Raviele A, Natale A, Calkins H, et al. Venice Chart international consensus document on atrial fibrillation ablation: 2011 update. J Cardiovasc Electrophysiol 2012;23(8):890–923.

18. Santangeli P, Zado ES, Hutchinson MD, et al. Prevalence and distribution of focal triggers in persistent and long-standing persistent atrial fibrillation. Heart Rhythm 2016;13(2):374–82.

19. Gokoglan Y, Mohanty S, Gunes MF, et al. Pulmonary vein antrum isolation in patients with paroxysmal atrial fibrillation: more than a decade of follow-up. Circ Arrhythm Electrophysiol 2016;9(5) [pii: e003660].

20. Blom NA, Gittenberger-de Groot AC, DeRuiter MC, et al. Development of the cardiac conduction tissue in human embryos using HNK-1 antigen expression: possible relevance for understanding of abnormal atrial automaticity. Circulation 1999;99(6):800–6.

21. DeSimone CV, Noheria A, Lachman N, et al. Myocardium of the superior vena cava, coronary sinus, vein of Marshall, and the pulmonary vein ostia: gross anatomic studies in 620 hearts. J Cardiovasc Electrophysiol 2012;23(12):1304–9.

22. Patterson E, Lazzara R, Szabo B, et al. Sodium-calcium exchange initiated by the Ca2+ transient: an arrhythmia trigger within pulmonary veins. J Am Coll Cardiol 2006;47(6):1196–206.

23. Hocini M, Ho SY, Kawara T, et al. Electrical conduction in canine pulmonary veins: electrophysiological and anatomic correlation. Circulation 2002;105(20):2442–8.

24. Gianni C, Mohanty S, Trivedi C, et al. Novel concepts and approaches in ablation of atrial fibrillation: the role of non-pulmonary vein triggers. Europace 2018;20(10):1566–76.

25. Mohanty S, Mohanty P, Di Biase L, et al. Long-term follow-up of patients with paroxysmal atrial fibrillation and severe left atrial scarring: comparison between pulmonary vein antrum isolation only or pulmonary vein isolation combined with either scar homogenization or trigger ablation. Europace 2017;19(11):1790–7.

26. Patel D, Mohanty P, Di Biase L, et al. Outcomes and complications of catheter ablation for atrial fibrillation in females. Heart Rhythm 2010;7(2):167–72.

27. Mohanty S, Mohanty P, Di Biase L, et al. Impact of metabolic syndrome on procedural outcomes in patients with atrial fibrillation undergoing catheter ablation. J Am Coll Cardiol 2012;59(14):1295–301.

28. Patel D, Mohanty P, Di Biase L. Safety and efficacy of pulmonary vein antral isolation in patients with obstructive sleep apnea: the impact of continuous positive airway pressure. Circ Arrhythm Electrophysiol 2010;3(5):445–51.

29. Santangeli P, Di Biase L, Mohanty P, et al. Catheter ablation of atrial fibrillation in octogenarians: safety and outcomes. J Cardiovasc Electrophysiol 2012; 23(7):687–93.

30. Zhao Y, Di Biase L, Trivedi C, et al. Importance of non-pulmonary vein triggers ablation to achieve long-term freedom from paroxysmal atrial fibrillation in patients with low ejection fraction. Heart Rhythm 2016;13(1):141–9.

31. Verma A, Wazni OM, Marrouche NF, et al. Pre-existent left atrial scarring in patients undergoing pulmonary vein antrum isolation: an independent predictor of procedural failure. J Am Coll Cardiol 2005;45(2): 285–92.

32. Santangeli P, Di Biase L, Themistoclakis S, et al. Catheter ablation of atrial fibrillation in hypertrophic cardiomyopathy: long-term outcomes and mechanisms of arrhythmia recurrence. Circ Arrhythm Electrophysiol 2013;6(6):1089–94.

33. Bai R, Di Biase L, Mohanty P, et al. Catheter ablation of atrial fibrillation in patients with mechanical mitral valve: long-term outcome of single procedure of pulmonary vein antrum isolation with or without nonpulmonary vein trigger ablation. J Cardiovasc Electrophysiol 2014;25(8):824–33.

34. Anselmino M, Matta M, D' Ascenzo F, et al. Catheter ablation of atrial fibrillation in patients with diabetes mellitus: a systematic review and meta-analysis. Europace 2015;17(10):1518–25.

35. Santangeli P, Marchlinski FE. Techniques for the provocation, localization, and ablation of non-pulmonary vein triggers for atrial fibrillation. Heart Rhythm 2017;14(7):1087–96.

36. Abdulla R, Blew GA, Holterman MJ. Cardiovascular embryology. Pediatr Cardiol 2004;25(3):191–200.

37. Rohr S. Arrhythmogenic implications of fibroblast-myocyte interactions. Circ Arrhythm Electrophysiol 2012;5(2):442–52.

38. Wilber DJ. Fibroblasts, focal triggers, and persistent atrial fibrillation: is there a connection? Circ Arrhythm Electrophysiol 2012;5(2):249–51.

39. Platonov PG, Mitrofanova LB, Orshanskaya V, et al. Structural abnormalities in atrial walls are associated with presence and persistency of atrial fibrillation but not with age. J Am Coll Cardiol 2011;58(21): 2225–32.

40. Suenari K, Di Biase L, Mohanty P, et al. Discrepant electrophysiological characteristics and calcium homeostasis of left atrial anterior and posterior myocytes. Basic Res Cardiol 2011;106(1):65–74.

41. Bai R, Di Biase L, Mohanty P, et al. Proven isolation of the pulmonary vein antrum with or without left atrial posterior wall isolation in patients with persistent atrial fibrillation. Heart Rhythm 2016;13(1): 132–40.

42. He X, Zhou Y, Chen Y, et al. Left atrial posterior wall isolation reduces the recurrence of atrial fibrillation: a meta-analysis. J Interv Card Electrophysiol 2016; 46(3):267–74.

43. Sanders P, Hocini M, Jais P, et al. Complete isolation of the pulmonary veins and posterior left atrium in chronic atrial fibrillation. Long-term clinical outcome. Eur Heart J 2007;28(15):1862–71.

44. Kim JS, Shin SY, Na JO, et al. Does isolation of the left atrial posterior wall improve clinical outcomes after radiofrequency catheter ablation for persistent atrial fibrillation?: a prospective randomized clinical trial. Int J Cardiol 2015;181:277–83.

45. McLellan AJA, Prabhu S, Voskoboinik A, et al. Isolation of the posterior left atrium for patients with persistent atrial fibrillation: routine adenosine challenge for dormant posterior left atrial conduction improves long-term outcome. Europace 2017;19(12): 1958–66.

46. Lupercio F, Lin AY, Aldaas OM, et al. Role of adjunctive posterior wall isolation in patients undergoing atrial fibrillation ablation: a systematic review and meta-analysis. J Interv Card Electrophysiol 2019. [Epub ahead of print].

47. Tamborero D, Mont L, Berruezo A, et al. Left atrial posterior wall isolation does not improve the outcome of circumferential pulmonary vein ablation for atrial fibrillation: a prospective randomized study. Circ Arrhythm Electrophysiol 2009;2(1):35–40.

48. Verma A, Kilicaslan F, Adams JR, et al. Extensive ablation during pulmonary vein antrum isolation has no adverse impact on left atrial function: an echocardiography and cine computed tomography analysis. J Cardiovasc Electrophysiol 2006;17(7):741–6.

49. Aryana A, Baker JH, Espinosa Ginic MA, et al. Posterior wall isolation using the cryoballoon in conjunction with pulmonary vein ablation is superior to pulmonary vein isolation alone in patients with persistent atrial fibrillation: a multicenter experience. Heart Rhythm 2018;15(8):1121–9.

50. Arruda M, Mlcochova H, Prasad SK, et al. Electrical isolation of the superior vena cava: an adjunctive strategy to pulmonary vein antrum isolation improving the outcome of AF ablation. J Cardiovasc Electrophysiol 2007;18(12):1261–6.

51. Tsai CF, Tai CT, Hsieh MH, et al. Initiation of atrial fibrillation by ectopic beats originating from the superior vena cava: electrophysiological characteristics and results of radiofrequency ablation. Circulation 2000;102(1):67–74.

52. Huang BH, Wu MH, Tsao HM, et al. Morphology of the thoracic veins and left atrium in paroxysmal atrial fibrillation initiated by superior caval vein ectopy. J Cardiovasc Electrophysiol 2005;16(4):411–7.

53. Ejima K, Kato K, Iwanami Y, et al. Impact of an empiric isolation of the superior vena cava in addition to circumferential pulmonary vein isolation on the outcome of paroxysmal atrial fibrillation ablation. Am J Cardiol 2015;116(11):1711–6.

54. Corrado A, Bonso A, Madalosso M, et al. Impact of systematic isolation of superior vena cava in addition to pulmonary vein antrum isolation on the outcome of paroxysmal, persistent, and permanent atrial fibrillation ablation: results from a randomized study. J Cardiovasc Electrophysiol 2010;21(1):1–5.

55. Yoshiga Y, Shimizu A, Ueyama T, et al. Strict sequential catheter ablation strategy targeting the pulmonary veins and superior vena cava for persistent atrial fibrillation. J Cardiol 2018;72(2):128–34.

56. Della Rocca DG, Mohanty S, Mohanty P, et al. Long-term outcomes of catheter ablation in patients with longstanding persistent atrial fibrillation lasting less than 2 years. J Cardiovasc Electrophysiol 2018;29(12):1607–15.

57. Xu K, Wang Y, Wu S, et al. The role of superior vena cava in catheter ablation of long-standing persistent atrial fibrillation. Europace 2017;19(10):1670–5.

58. Gianni C, Sanchez JE, Mohanty S, et al. Isolation of the superior vena cava from the right atrial posterior wall: a novel ablation approach. Europace 2018; 20(9):e124–32.

59. Oral H, Ozaydin M, Chugh A, et al. Role of the coronary sinus in maintenance of atrial fibrillation. J Cardiovasc Electrophysiol 2003;14(12):1329–36.

60. Haissaguerre M, Hocini M, Takahashi Y, et al. Impact of catheter ablation of the coronary sinus on paroxysmal or persistent atrial fibrillation. J Cardiovasc Electrophysiol 2007;18(4):378–86.

61. Knecht S, O' Neill MD, Matsuo S, et al. Focal arrhythmia confined within the coronary sinus and maintaining atrial fibrillation. J Cardiovasc Electrophysiol 2007;18(11):1140–6.

62. Chang HY, Lo LW, Lin YJ, et al. Long-term outcome of catheter ablation in patients with atrial fibrillation originating from nonpulmonary vein ectopy. J Cardiovasc Electrophysiol 2013;24(3):250–8.

63. Chauvin M, Shah DC, Haissaguerre M, et al. The anatomic basis of connections between the coronary sinus musculature and the left atrium in humans. Circulation 2000;101(6):647–52.

64. Ho SY, Sanchez-Quintana D, Becker AE. A review of the coronary venous system: a road less travelled. Heart Rhythm 2004;1(1):107–12.

65. Morita H, Zipes DP, Morita ST, et al. Isolation of canine coronary sinus musculature from the atria by radiofrequency catheter ablation prevents induction of atrial fibrillation. Circ Arrhythm Electrophysiol 2014;7(6):1181–8.

66. Yin X, Zhao Z, Gao L, et al. Frequency gradient within coronary sinus predicts the long-term outcome of persistent atrial fibrillation catheter ablation. J Am Heart Assoc 2017;6(3) [pii: e004869].

67. Gunes MF, Gokoglan Y, Di Biase L, et al. Ablating the posterior heart: cardioesophageal fistula complicating radiofrequency ablation in the coronary sinus. J Cardiovasc Electrophysiol 2015;26(12):1376–8.

68. Di Biase L, Burkhardt JD, Mohanty P, et al. Left atrial appendage: an underrecognized trigger site of atrial fibrillation. Circulation 2010;122(2):109–18.

69. Hocini M, Shah AJ, Nault I, et al. Localized reentry within the left atrial appendage: arrhythmogenic role in patients undergoing ablation of persistent atrial fibrillation. Heart Rhythm 2011;8(12): 1853–61.

70. Di Biase L, Burkhardt JD, Mohanty P, et al. Left atrial appendage isolation in patients with longstanding persistent AF undergoing catheter ablation: BELIEF trial. J Am Coll Cardiol 2016;68(18):1929–40.

71. Friedman DJ, Black-Maier EW, Barnett AS, et al. Left atrial appendage electrical isolation for treatment of recurrent atrial fibrillation: a meta-analysis. JACC Clin Electrophysiol 2018;4(1):112–20.

72. Romero J, Michaud GF, Avendano R, et al. Benefit of left atrial appendage electrical isolation for persistent and long-standing persistent atrial fibrillation: a systematic review and meta-analysis. Europace 2018;20(8):1268–78.

73. Rillig A, Tilz RR, Lin T, et al. Unexpectedly high incidence of stroke and left atrial appendage thrombus formation after electrical isolation of the left atrial appendage for the treatment of atrial tachyarrhythmias. Circ Arrhythm Electrophysiol 2016;9(5): e003461.

74. Briceno DF, Di Biase L, Natale A. Letter from Briceno et al regarding article, "an unexpectedly high incidence of stroke and left atrial appendage thrombus formation after electrical isolation of the left atrial appendage for the treatment of atrial tachyarrhythmias". Circ Arrhythm Electrophysiol 2016;9(9) [pii: e004485].

75. Di Biase L, Mohanty S, Trivedi C, et al. Stroke risk in patients with atrial fibrillation undergoing electrical isolation of the left atrial appendage. J Am Coll Cardiol 2019;74(8):1019–28.

76. Yorgun H, Canpolat U, Kocyigit D, et al. Left atrial appendage isolation in addition to pulmonary vein isolation in persistent atrial fibrillation: one-year clinical outcome after cryoballoon-based ablation. Europace 2017;19(5):758–68.

77. Dearstine M, Taylor W, Kerut EK. Persistent left superior vena cava: chest x-ray and echocardiographic findings. Echocardiography 2000;17(5):453–5.

78. Turagam MK, Atoui M, Atkins D, et al. Persistent left superior vena cava as an arrhythmogenic source in atrial fibrillation: results from a multicenter experience. J Interv Card Electrophysiol 2019;54(2): 93–100.

79. Kim YG, Han S, Choi JI, et al. Impact of persistent left superior vena cava on radiofrequency catheter

ablation in patients with atrial fibrillation. Europace 2019 [pii:euz254].

80. Gonna H, Domenichini G, Conti S, et al. Cryoballoon isolation of the superior vena cava. JACC Clin Electrophysiol 2016;2(4):529–31.

81. Santoro F, Rillig A, Sohns C, et al. Second-generation cryoballoon atrial fibrillation ablation in patients with persistent left superior caval vein. JACC Clin Electrophysiol 2019;5(5):590–8.

82. Fujino T, Yuzawa H, Kinoshita T, et al. A case of successful cryoballoon ablation of paroxysmal atrial fibrillation originating from a persistent left superior vena cava. J Cardiol Cases 2019;20(3):77–80.

83. Briceno DF, Valderrabano M. Recurrent perimitral flutter due to vein of Marshall epicardial connections bypassing the mitral isthmus: response to ethanol infusion. Circ Arrhythm Electrophysiol 2014;7(5):988–9.

84. Kurotobi T, Ito H, Inoue K, et al. Marshall vein as arrhythmogenic source in patients with atrial fibrillation: correlation between its anatomy and electrophysiological findings. J Cardiovasc Electrophysiol 2006;17(10):1062–7.

85. Dave AS, Baez-Escudero JL, Sasaridis C, et al. Role of the vein of Marshall in atrial fibrillation recurrences after catheter ablation: therapeutic effect of ethanol infusion. J Cardiovasc Electrophysiol 2012;23(6):583–91.

86. Rodriguez-Manero M, Schurmann P, Valderrabano M. Ligament and vein of Marshall: a therapeutic opportunity in atrial fibrillation. Heart Rhythm 2016;13(2):593–601.

87. Chugh A, Gurm HS, Krishnasamy K, et al. Spectrum of atrial arrhythmias using the ligament of Marshall in patients with atrial fibrillation. Heart Rhythm 2018;15(1):17–24.

Fluoroless Atrial Fibrillation Catheter Ablation
Technique and Clinical Outcomes

Jorge Romero, MD[a], Kavisha Patel, MD[a], David Briceno, MD[a], Isabella Alviz, MD[a], Nicola Tarantino, MD[a], Domenico G. Della Rocca, MD[b], Veronica Natale, BS[b], Xiao-Dong Zhang, MD[a], Luigi Di Biase, MD, PhD, FHRS[a,*]

KEYWORDS

- Fluoroless • Ablation • Atrial fibrillation • Technique • Outcomes • Radiation
- Intracardiac echocardiography

KEY POINTS

- Most electrophysiology laboratories worldwide continue to use fluoroscopy routinely during catheter ablation (CA) for atrial fibrillation (AF).
- With increasing volume and complexity of AF ablation worldwide, the detrimental effects of radiation exposure to patients, physicians, and catheter laboratory staff are gaining increased consideration.
- Complete elimination or maximal reduction of fluoroscopy use has been reported in supraventricular tachycardia and right-sided accessory pathway ablation; however, CA for AF is a more complex procedure.
- This article describes an approach to fluoroless AF ablation and summarizes outcomes of studies evaluating zero to near-zero fluoroscopy use.
- Training electrophysiologists to gain more experience with intracardiac echocardiography as the primary imaging modality to perform transseptal access and to assess real-time lesion formation during ablation.

INTRODUCTION

The concept of fluoroless atrial fibrillation (AF) ablation was first introduced approximately a decade ago.[1] Despite the availability of intracardiac echocardiography (ICE), and growing use of electroanatomic mapping (EAM) systems, both reliable visual modalities to perform transseptal and confirm catheter positioning and movement, respectively. Fluoroscopy continues to be considered an indispensable part of the procedure for most electrophysiologists. Worldwide adoption of catheter ablation (CA) as the standard therapy for symptomatic AF, better understanding of arrhythmia substrates, and technological advancements have led to an exponential increase in the number and complexity of AF ablation procedures in recent years. Along with this upsurge, the detrimental effects of radiation exposure to patients, physicians, and catheter laboratory staff[2–7] are now gaining increased consideration. Exposure to ionizing

Funding: This research did not receive any funding.
[a] Montefiore Medical Center, Albert Einstein College of Medicine, 111 East 210th Street, Bronx, NY 10467, USA; [b] Texas Cardiac Arrhythmia Institute, St. David's Medical Center, Austin, TX, USA
* Corresponding author.
E-mail address: dibbia@gmail.com

cardiacEP.theclinics.com

radiation is known to result in 2 types of injury patterns: dose-dependent or deterministic (tissue reactions) injuries and non–dose-dependent or stochastic (carcinogenic, genetic effects) injuries. The dose-dependent injuries include skin erythema and cataracts; the non–dose-dependent injuries include malignancy and birth defects.[8–13]

A single procedure of AF ablation typically involves a high median dose of radiation exposure (~16.6 mSv); (range: 6.6–59.2 mSv).[14,15] This dose is roughly equivalent to the radiation dose received from 830 chest radiographs or 6.9 years of background radiation exposure.[14,15] This exposure is compounded by the need for repeat procedures in 15% to 50% of recurrent AF cases. The need for preprocedural computed tomography (CT) imaging to improve delineation of the pulmonary veins (PVs) and the left atrium (LA) anatomy also adds to this. The amount of ionizing radiation exposure to patients is extremely high, especially when 64-slice multidetector CT and electrocardiogram (ECG)-gating protocols with or without tube current modulation are used (i.e., 9mSv and 15 mSv, respectively).[16] Furthermore, obese patients are at higher risk, because they tend to receive twice the radiation exposure compared with average-sized patients,[17] leading to 2.5 times the lifetime risk of cancer-related mortality.[17] At inception, mean fluoroscopy duration during AF ablation was reported to be more than 60 minutes, which is equivalent to 4-fold the radiation exposure to patients undergoing CA for atrial flutter and supraventricular tachycardia (SVT).[18] For patients, this conferred a predicted excess risk of fatal malignancies of 0.07% and 0.1% in women and men, respectively.[18] For professionals, the excess lifetime cancer risk is estimated at 1 in 100 operators.[19] A recent report noted a higher risk of development of brain tumors in physicians performing interventional procedures.[20] A causal relation to occupational radiation exposure was suggested, given a disproportionate amount of left-sided tumors, because the head is relatively unprotected, and there is more radiation exposure to the left brain than the right.[20] A survey of interventional cardiologists and radiologists using lead attire reported that ~50% have spine problems and 25% have issues related to hip, knee, or ankle.[13]

Lately, there has been significant emphasis on reduction in radiation exposure via decrease in fluoroscopy time. Additional measures to decrease radiation exposure include reduction in frame rate, image intensity, and maximal collimation use.[21] The objective is to use radiation dose in accordance with the ALARA (as low as reasonably achievable) principle.[13] Complete elimination

of fluoroscopy use was initially reported in pediatric cases involving CA of right-sided accessory pathways and SVT.[22–24] Furthermore, ablation of left-sided pathways has been reported, with transseptal access being performed solely under transesophageal echocardiogram (TEE) guidance.[25] In adults, routine use of TEE to perform transseptal access is not a realistic alternative. Also, CA for AF is a more complex procedure compared with CA for an accessory pathway or atrial flutter. Most electrophysiologists have been trained to use fluoroscopy as the principal imaging modality to perform transseptal puncture and are hesitant about substituting it with ICE. The main hurdle to the adoption of a completely fluoroless approach to AF ablation has been a lack of preparedness to abandon an old practice. Nonetheless, this can be remediated by increasing knowledge, familiarity, training, and experience in this method. Although associated with a steep learning curve, the skillset can be willingly acquired. It is fair to state that minimal fluoroscopy could be considered a viable alternative option.

TECHNIQUE

Accurate three-dimensional (3D) reconstruction of the LA and PVs is a crucial step in effective and safe AF radiofrequency (RF) ablation. The proposed techniques to implement this include ICE,[26,27] fast anatomic mapping (FAM), and EAM.[28] The ultrasonography-based 3D imaging system (CARTOSound, Biosense Webster Inc, Diamond Bar, CA)[29,30] permits integration of serial two-dimensional (2D) LA sector scans obtained from the ICE catheter placed in the right atrium (RA). Quick real-time creation of the LA anatomy using FAM can be achieved by using sensor-based catheters in the LA. These methods can be used alone or in combination with preacquired CT or MRI scans. The authors recommend merging 2D phased array ICE with CT or MRI. Alternatively, 3D ICE-based images can be combined with FAM and/or EAM (**Fig. 1**).

During AF ablation, the use of fluoroscopy has been thought to be fundamental for the following steps: (1) catheter advancement into the coronary sinus (CS), (2) advancement of guidewires and sheaths into the superior vena cava (SVC), (3) performing transseptal puncture (TSP), and advancement of sheaths and catheters into the LA. Once a multipolar mapping catheter (MMC) and ablation catheter are advanced into the LA, most electrophysiologists are comfortable without the use of fluoroscopy. This article describes fluoroless techniques to safely execute these steps.

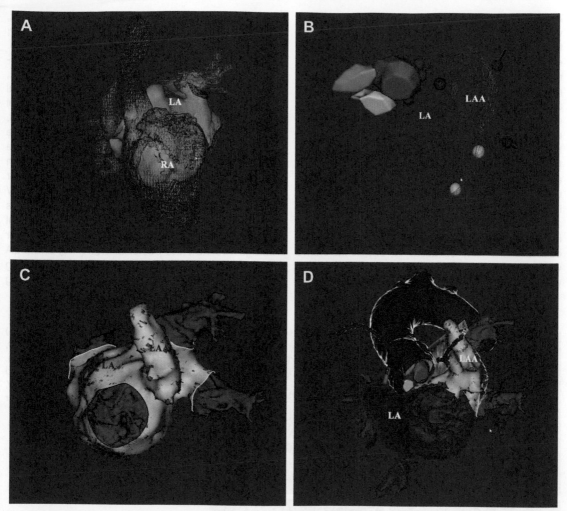

Fig. 1. Integration of multiple imaging modalities. (*A*) RA was reconstructed using the preprocedural CT scan, and the LA was reconstructed with FAM. (*B, C*) CARTOSound anatomic map based on ICE shows delineation of the LA, PVs, and left atrial appendage (LAA); (*D*) Imaging integration with CARTOSound, FAM, and 3D CT scan.

Ultrasonography-Guided Vascular Access

The common femoral veins can be easily accessed via the groin. A high-frequency linear transducer (5–10 MHz) is used because it allows better resolution of tissues close to the skin surface. On ultrasonography, the lumen of a vessel appears black, whereas the surrounding tissue appears some level of gray. Veins are oval or circular, thin-walled structures, and are easily compressed with light pressure. The common femoral vein is located medial to the common femoral artery. It is important to orient the ultrasonography probe correctly. By convention, left-sided structures beneath the probe should be displayed on the left side of the imaging screen, which also allows better intuitive sense for needle movement for the operator. The Seldinger technique is used to obtain vascular access. The center of the vein is targeted on transverse view; once the needle tip crosses the skin, negative pressure is applied on the syringe while advancing the needle. Blood return is noted when the venous endothelium is punctured. The needle is stabilized in place, the syringe is removed, and a guidewire is introduced into the vein. It is crucial to confirm the position of the guidewire in transverse and longitudinal axes before the sheaths are advanced.

Navigating the Intracardiac Echocardiography Catheter

A phased array ICE catheter (8 or 10 French) is inserted through the left femoral vein. The elementary rule for safe advancement of the ICE catheter is to continuously maintain a long-axis view of the vein; an experienced operator can easily advance this to the RA without the use of fluoroscopy. An echocardiographic clear space (black) should be maintained in front of the catheter during advancement, and the operator should avoid pushing when an echogenic space (white) is seen. The ICE catheter offers a depth of penetration of up to 15 cm and can be deflected in 4 positions (anterior/posterior and left/right). The transducer is present on the tip of the catheter; ICE images are presented as 90° sectors originating from the transducer, with the image sector being perpendicular to the long axis of the catheter. In cases where initial advancement of the ICE probe from the iliac veins into the inferior vena cava is challenging, long access sheaths may be used. To obtain the home view, the ICE catheter is placed in the mid-RA, with the transducer in neutral position, facing the

tricuspid valve. It provides a view of the RA, tricuspid valve, the right ventricle (RV) and, usually, a longitudinal axis view of the aortic valve (**Fig. 2**A). Gentle rotation of the ICE catheter clockwise (posteriorly) helps visualize the interatrial septum, RA, LA, LV, and the CS os (**Fig. 2**B). The left atrial appendage can also be visualized at this level (**Fig. 2**C). CS os is annotated using CARTOSound. The catheter is then rotated further clockwise (posteriorly) until the left upper and lower PVs are in view; they often appear as a pair of pants with a common ostium (**Fig. 2**D). Often, the left superior PV comes into view before the left inferior PV because it is a more anterior structure. These veins are then marked on CARTOSound. Additional clockwise/posterior rotation of the ICE catheter brings into view the posterior wall (PW) of the LA and the esophagus along its long axis. Marking the outline of the esophagus aids in integrating

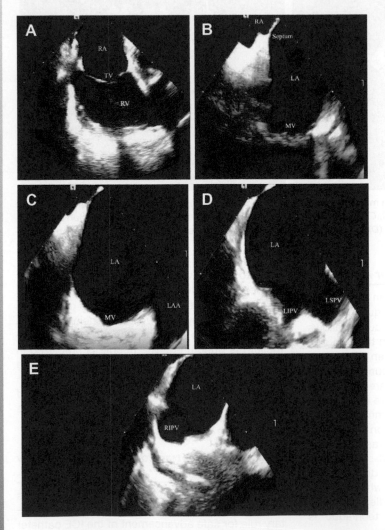

Fig. 2. (*A–E*) Basic ICE views. (*A*) Home view: RA, tricuspid valve (TV), and the RV. (*B*) Interatrial septum, RA, LA. (*C*) LAA. (*D*) Left upper and lower PVs. (*E*) Right inferior PV. LIPV, left inferior PV; LSPV, left superior PV; MV, mitral valve.

its location on FAM/EAM and CT/MRI later. It is important to accurately determine esophageal location and its course in relation to PVs to avoid injury to it at the time of RF energy delivery. More clockwise/posterior torque and slight advancement of the ICE catheter brings into view the right inferior (7 o'clock) (**Fig. 2**E) and right superior PVs (5 o'clock), respectively.

Advancing coronary sinus catheter

Next, if a CS catheter is needed, this can be introduced from the left femoral vein. The authors suggest using a 7 french F curve catheter (DECANAV, Biosense Webster Inc, Diamond Bar, CA), which permits direct visualization of the catheter as it is advanced toward the CS os (marked on CT or 3D ICE image) (**Fig. 3**). Likewise, this catheter allows for FAM of this structure.

Advancing guidewire/sheath into the superior vena cava for transseptal puncture

Before performance of transseptal puncture, a heparin bolus is administered, followed by a continuous infusion with a target activated clotting time between 350 and 400 seconds. ICE allows optimum visualization of the junction of the RA and SVC to direct advancement of guidewires and sheaths. From the home view, the ICE

catheter is gently rotated clockwise (posteriorly) until the interatrial septum is visualized along with fossa ovalis (**Fig. 4**). Further posterior tilt and rightward flexion is provided to visualize the SVC. Subsequently, a 180-cm long J-tipped wire (0.8 mm [0.032 inches]) is introduced via the right femoral vein (see **Fig. 4**A). A steerable transseptal sheath (8.5 French) and dilator are then advanced over the guidewire under direct visualization by ICE, confirming that the tip of the guidewire is always distal to the tip of the dilator (see **Fig. 4**B). Once the sheath is in the SVC (see **Fig. 4**C), the guidewire is exchanged for the Brockenbrough transseptal needle. The needle is advanced and positioned proximal to the tip of the dilator with a space of 2 fingerbreadths between the needle hub and the sheath.

Performance of transseptal puncture

The complete equipment is then slowly pulled back from the SVC and directed posteriorly. Simultaneously, the posterior torque on the ICE catheter is released until the interatrial septum and fossa ovalis are visualized. The aim is to tent the center of the fossa ovalis with the dilator sheath, ideally with left-sided PVs in view (**Fig. 5**A). It is important to avoid tenting very anteriorly in order to prevent injury to the aortic root. In

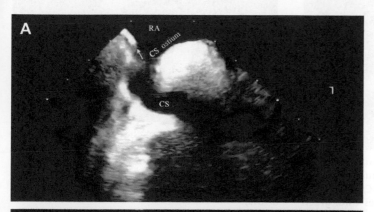
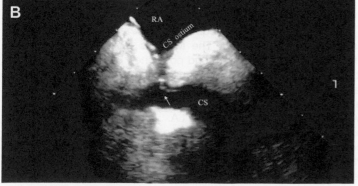

Fig. 3. Advancing CS catheter. (*A*) Decapolar catheter is at the ostium of the CS; (*B*) the catheter is advanced into the CS. Yellow arrow indicates the tip of the catheter.

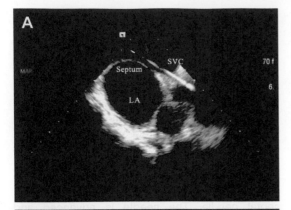

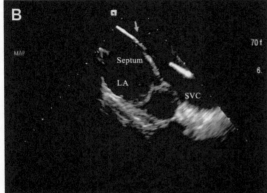

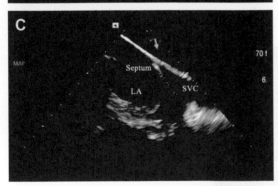

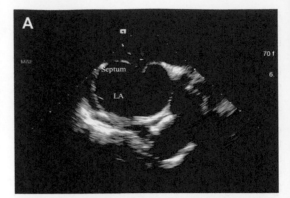

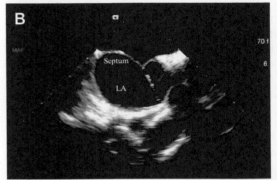

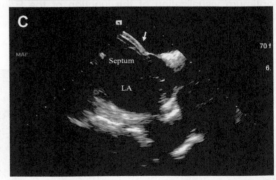

Fig. 5. (*A–C*) TSP: (*A*) tent the center of fossa ovalis with the dilator sheath (*red arrow*); (*B*) needle is slowly advanced to puncture the fossa ovalis (*red arrow*); (*C*) needle position is stabilized, dilator and sheath are advanced to cover the needle (*white arrow*).

Fig. 4. (*A, B*) Interatrial septum is visualized along with fossa ovalis and SVC; (*A*) guidewire; (*B*) advancing guidewire/sheaths into SVC; (*C*) sheath advanced into SVC. Red arrow indicates wire; green arrow indicates sheath.

contrast, tenting too posteriorly can increase the risk of damage to the PW of the LA. Once an optimum tenting site is confirmed on ICE, the needle is slowly advanced to puncture the fossa ovalis. The authors usually use the SafeSept wire to facilitate this step and avoid risk of lateral LA wall perforation (**Fig. 5**B). Following this, needle position is stabilized; dilator and sheath are advanced over this wire to cover the needle (**Fig. 5**C). After ensuring that the dilator is not touching the lateral LA wall, the sheath is advanced over the dilator into the

LA. Subsequently, the needle and dilator are removed. The MMC is then advanced through the sheath and positioned in the left superior PV. The exact technique is repeated for the second transseptal access if needed, and the ablation catheter is then advanced through the second sheath into the LA.

It is common to experience resistance while trying to advance the dilator and sheath given the step-up in diameter. This resistance can commonly be resolved by gentle clockwise and counterclockwise rotation of the sheath while advancing it from the RA into the LA. In difficult cases with anatomic alterations in septum (thickness, elasticity, size, or aneurysm), an RF transseptal needle, connected to an RF generator (Baylis Medical Company, Montreal, Canada), can be used to puncture the fossa ovalis. In the TRAVERSE LA (Randomized Trial of Conventional Transseptal Needle Versus Radiofrequency Energy Needle Puncture for Left Atrial Access) study, the efficacy and safety of this technique was similar to conventional needle puncture with a shorter transseptal puncture time and less frequent plastic shavings with the RF needle.[31] The proposed mechanism for the use of RF energy for transseptal puncture is via electrically charged fragments that create a pore in the myocyte membrane.[32] Subsequent local increase in temperature causes evaporation of water in the cells in front of the needle tip, leading to limited tissue desiccation.[33]

Tracking of transseptal sheath

In cases where transseptal access is unintentionally lost, the sheath can be reintroduced into the LA without the use of fluoroscopy. Acquiring anatomy of the RA at the time of insertion of the ablation catheter and annotating this site on FAM/CT image can aid in performing this step. Earlier, the tip of the transseptal sheath could not be determined on FAM. However, its position can be determined indirectly by advancing and retracting the sheath over the ablation catheter. While using CARTO (Biosense Webster Inc, Diamond Bar, CA), the shaft of the ablation catheter has 2 proximal electrodes, which are located 43 mm and 72 mm away from the tip, respectively. On the distal aspect of the catheter, 4 electrodes are present (16 mm from the tip). System patches process the signal from these electrodes. Based on the degree of advancement of the ablation catheter in relation to the sheath, the shaft and curvature of the catheter are visualized. When all the electrodes are covered, an alert "SH" (sheath) appears on the monitor. Recently, the VIZIGO Bi-directional Guiding Sheath (Biosense Webster Inc, Diamond Bar, CA) was introduced, which allows direct sheath visualization on the CARTO mapping system (Fig. 6).

Left atrium mapping and radiofrequency energy delivery

Following the introduction of the MMC and ablation catheter into the LA, FAM/EAM can be used for precise 3D reconstruction of the LA and PVs. The MMC is then advanced into each of the PVs, and its position is confirmed on ICE and EAM. Wide circumferential RF lesions are then applied to achieve PV isolation (PVI) in patients with paroxysmal AF. The real-time lesion formation is assessed by ICE. In patients with persistent AF, more extensive ablation can be performed as deemed necessary (Fig. 7). The authors use Esophastar (Biosense Webster Inc, Diamond Bar, CA) (Fig. 8) to create an anatomic map of the esophagus; it creates a virtual esophageal tube using point-to-point mapping. Compared with CT, it provides real-time information and reconstructs a more precise esophageal image.[34] It can help determine the exact esophageal location in relation to the ablation sites as necessary for accurate assessment of esophageal temperatures when RF energy is delivered, and provides a reliable alternative to fluoroscopy use. In general, most electrophysiologists are comfortable performing this portion of AF ablation without the use of fluoroscopy.

CLINICAL OUTCOMES

Efforts to minimize or completely relinquish fluoroscopy use during AF ablation have been directed toward 2 broad categories: before/during and after TSP. The former has been more challenging to achieve, because it requires training electrophysiologists to rely on ICE for performing TSP, an undertaking that has heavily relied on fluoroscopic guidance in the past. The latter has been easier to execute with the incorporation of newer nonfluoroscopic mapping systems into routine clinical practice. Integration of nonfluoroscopic catheter visualization technology (NFCV) and 3D EAM allows operators to manipulate mapping and ablation catheters in a fluoroscopic environment without the use of live fluoroscopy. Huo and colleagues,[35] conducted the first prospective, randomized trial to assess the benefit of a novel fluoroscopy image integrated EAM (F-EAM) system (CARTO 3 with the UNIVU module, Biosense Webster, Inc, Diamond Bar, CA) compared with the conventional EAM system (CARTO 3, Biosense Webster). Eighty patients with paroxysmal AF were randomized in a 1:1 fashion to F-EAM or EAM arms. With the use of the F-EAM system, both fluoroscopy time and radiation exposure were significantly lower (1 minute 45 seconds, interquartile range [IQR] 1 minute 5 seconds to 2 minutes 22 seconds; vs 10 minutes 42 seconds, IQR, 18 minutes 45 seconds to 12 minutes 46 seconds, $P<.001$; 652 cGy cm^2 vs 2440 cGy cm^2, $P<.001$). Overall, a striking 73% decrease in radiation doses and 84% reduction in fluoroscopy time were achieved with the F-EAM system compared with the EAM system. Importantly, this was achieved with no

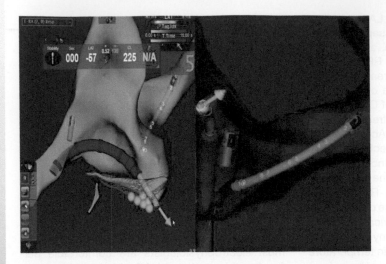

Fig. 6. VIZIGO Bi-directional Guiding Sheath can be visualized on EAM.

added procedural time (F-EAM, 1 hour 37 minutes, IQR, 1 hour 17 minutes to 1 hour 50 minutes; vs EAM, 1 hour 39 minutes, IQR, 1 hour 18 minutes to 2 hours 10 minutes; P = nonsignificant [NS]), and no significant difference in arrhythmia-free survival rates between the 2 groups (F-EAM 72.5%vs EAM 80%, P = NS). Sommer and colleagues,[36] in a cohort of 375 consecutive patients, assessed a different fluoroscopy integrated sensor–based tracking technology (MediGuide, St. Jude Medical Inc, St Paul, MN) and EAM system (EnSite Velocity, St. Jude Medical Inc, St Paul, MN). When the initial 50 cases were compared with the last 50 cases, fluoroscopy time reduced from 6 minutes (IQR, 4.1–10.3 minutes) to 1.1 minutes (IQR, 0.7–1.5 minutes); radiation dose decreased from 2363 cGy cm² to 490 cGy cm². Mean procedural

time of ~135 minutes and complication rate of ~2.7% were reported. In the largest real-world study[37] to date, comprising 1000 patients undergoing AF ablation, use of NFCV technology resulted in a median procedure time of 120 minutes, median fluoroscopy time of 0.9 minutes, and median fluoroscopy dose of 345 cGy cm². Successful PVI was accomplished in 99.9% cases with an overall complication rate of ~2%. These studies[35–37] report reduction in fluoroscopy use almost exclusively after TSP.

A decade ago, the first report on complete elimination of fluoroscopy for AF ablation was published.[1] In 19 out of 21 patients with AF, fluoroless AF ablation was successfully completed. Although the safety and feasibility of this approach was recognized, median procedure time was considerably high (208 minutes). A year

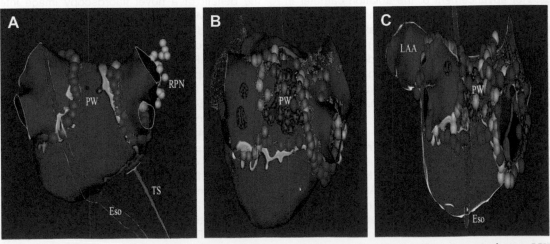

Fig. 7. (A) PV isolation; (B) PV plus PW isolation, (C) PV plus PW plus LAA electrical isolation. Eso, esophagus; RPN, right phrenic nerve.

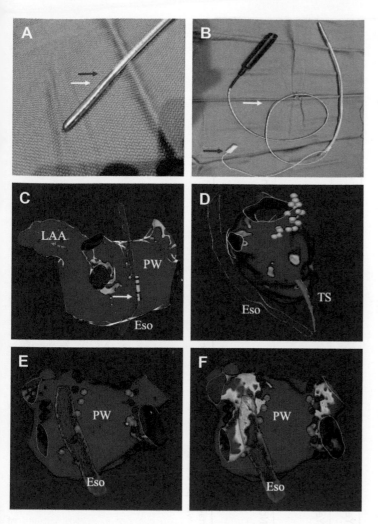

Fig. 8. (*A, B*) Esophageal temperature probe with esophageal mapping catheter catheter is inserted inside the esophageal probe (*white arrow, esophageal mapping catheter; red arrow, esophageal probe*); (*C–F*) accurate esophageal dimensions are mapped using the this setup.

later, Reddy and colleagues,[38] reaffirmed the safety and efficacy of a fluoroless approach in another small study of 20 patients with paroxysmal AF. Although there were no complications, and electrical isolation was achieved in 97% of ipsilateral PV isolating lesion sets, the procedure time was again considerable (224 ± 75 minutes). Both of these studies[1,38] used a combination of ICE and the NavX EAM system (St. Jude Medical Inc, St Paul, MN) to confirm catheter positioning and movement. Five years after the initial report, Bulava and colleagues,[39] published the first randomized study on fluoroless CA for AF, integrating ICE and the CARTO 3 EAM system (Biosense Webster Inc, Diamond Bar, CA). The purpose of this study was to evaluate the impact of an important technological development in 3D mapping since the prior studies[1,38] (i.e., contact force measurement with SmartTouch technology). Eighty patients were randomized in a 1:1 fashion to PVI

under fluoroscopic guidance (X+) and PVI with zero fluoroscopy use (X−). For both X− and X+ groups, total procedural time and RF delivery time were similar (92.5 ± 22.9 minutes vs 99.9 ± 15.9 minutes, P = NS); (1785 ± 548 seconds vs 1755 ± 450 seconds, P = NS). In all except 1 patient in the X− group, 8 seconds of fluoroscopy was required to verify the position of the guidewire in the femoral vein. The complication rates and arrhythmia-free survival rates at 12 months of follow-up were similar between the 2 groups. In addition, a drastic reduction in total procedural time using a fluoroless approach was noted: 92 minutes versus 224 and 208 minutes in prior studies.[1,38] Liu and Palmer[40] published the largest series of fluoroless AF ablation to date, involving 200 patients with paroxysmal and persistent AF. Fluoroless AF ablation was effectively completed for the entire cohort, success rate was 76% at a mean follow-up of

Table 1
Summary of published studies on fluoroless atrial fibrillation ablation

Study Source	Number of Fluoroless AF Ablations	Mean Procedure Time (min)	Requirement of 3D Mapping for PVI	Persistent AF Inclusion	Zero Fluoroscopy (%)	Inclusion of Patients with PPM/ICD Leads	Complication Rate (%)
Ferguson et al,[1] 2009	21	208	Yes	Yes	90	No	0
Reddy et al,[38] 2010	20	244	Yes	No	100	No	0
Bulava et al,[39] 2015	40	92.5	Yes	No	97.5	No	0
Sanchez et al,[41] 2016	56	126	Yes	Yes	100	No	0
Percell et al,[42] 2016	20	210	Yes	Yes	95	No	5
Razminia et al,[43] 2017	186 (150 RF and 36 cryoballoon) over 5 y	194	Yes	Yes	99.5	No	1.6
Liu & Palmer,[40] 2018	200	90 for PVI only and 106 for the entire cohort	No	Yes	100	Yes (n = 19)	1

From Liu, X. and J. Palmer, Outcomes of 200 consecutive, fluoroless atrial fibrillation ablations using a new technique. Pacing Clin Electrophysiol, 2018. 41(11): p. 1404-1411. https://doi.org/10.1111/pace.13492. Copyright © 2018 Wiley Periodicals, Inc.; with permission.

11 months, and 2 complications occurred (right phrenic nerve palsy, right femoral artery pseudoaneurysm). Again, with the use of contact force technology, mean procedural time for PVI and the entire cohort (90.3 ± 17.7 minutes and 106.2 ± 23.2 minutes) were significantly better than in the initial studies.[1,38] Unlike prior studies,[1,38,39] 3D mapping for the entire LA was not performed. This study[40] was also the first to include patients with permanent pacemaker/implantable cardioverter-defibrillator (PPM/ICD) leads; interestingly, despite zero fluoroscopy use, AF ablation was successfully completed in all 19 patients without any reported lead dislodgement. **Table 1** summarizes a list of published studies on fluoroless AF ablation. All studies reported so far have used RF energy for AF ablation[1,38,39,41,42]; use of cryoballoon ablation for successful fluoroless AF ablation has only been reported in 30 cases by Razminia and colleagues.[42]

LIMITATIONS

Although appealing, it would be challenging to perform AF ablation without fluoroscopy in patients with atrial septal defect closure devices, poor ultrasonography windows, and anatomic abnormalities. More data are required before adopting a fluoroless approach in patients with PPM/ICD leads. The optimal patients for zero fluoroscopy use would be pregnant women and obese individuals. Concerns regarding need for a second operator to manipulate the ICE catheter have been raised, however, this is a small disadvantage, especially because this is necessary only until introduction of sheaths in the LA. Positioning the esophageal temperature probe is sometimes challenging with ICE. Anatomic mapping of the esophagus can be performed using Esophastar (Biosense Webster Inc, Diamond Bar, CA). When necessary, short sequences of fluoroscopy at lower frame rates and image intensity with maximal collimation can still be used.

FUTURE PERSPECTIVES

Radiation-diminishing techniques can be performed for preprocedural CT to delineate LA and PV anatomy. Preprocedural MRI use instead of CT scan can completely eliminate ionizing radiation exposure. Introduction of contact force sensors along the tip and body of the sheath can further assist a fluoroless approach. A location sensor on the tip of the esophageal probe might also be helpful while ablating the PW of the LA. A sensor on the tip of the RF transseptal needle is

already available. The VIZIGO Bi-directional Guiding Sheath now permits direct sheath visualization on EAM. Although this article is limited to the use of RF energy for AF ablation, cryoablation can also be performed using the same steps in a fluoroless manner. Because the transseptal sheath for cryoballoon ablation is much larger, use of a stiffer sheath can expedite puncture of the fossa ovalis.

SUMMARY

Fluoroless AF ablation and lead-free procedures in routine clinical practice have now become a realistic goal in most patients. The safety and efficacy of a fluoroless approach to AF ablation are similar to outcomes achieved with fluoroscopy use. Training electrophysiologists to gain more experience using ICE and EAM as the primary imaging modalities for AF ablation can help execute a fluoroless approach on a larger scale, minimizing the potential harms associated with ionizing radiation and lead attire.

DISCLOSURE

The authors have no disclosures related to this article.

REFERENCES

1. Ferguson JD, Helms A, Mangrum JM, et al. Catheter ablation of atrial fibrillation without fluoroscopy using intracardiac echocardiography and electroanatomic mapping. Circ Arrhythm Electrophysiol 2009;2:611–9.
2. Calkins H, Niklason L, Sousa J, et al. Radiation exposure during radiofrequency catheter ablation of accessory atrioventricular connections. Circulation 1991;84:2376–82.
3. Lindsay BD, Eichling JO, Ambos HD, et al. Radiation exposure to patients and medical personnel during radiofrequency catheter ablation for supraventricular tachycardia. Am J Cardiol 1992;70:218–23.
4. Kovoor P, Ricciardello M, Collins L, et al. Risk to patients from radiation associated with radiofrequency ablation for supraventricular tachycardia. Circulation 1998;98:1534–40.
5. Rosenthal LS, Mahesh M, Beck TJ, et al. Predictors of fluoroscopy time and estimated radiation exposure during radiofrequency catheter ablation procedures. Am J Cardiol 1998;82:451–8.
6. Perisinakis K, Damilakis J, Theocharopoulos N, et al. Accurate assessment of patient effective radiation dose and associated detriment risk from radiofrequency catheter ablation procedures. Circulation 2001;104:58–62.
7. Macle L, Weerasooriya R, Jais P, et al. Radiation exposure during radiofrequency catheter ablation

for atrial fibrillation. Pacing Clin Electrophysiol 2003; 26:288–91.

8. Rehani MM, Ortiz-Lopez P. Radiation effects in fluoroscopically guided cardiac interventions–keeping them under control. Int J Cardiol 2006;109:147–51.

9. Nahass GT. Fluoroscopy and the skin: implications for radiofrequency catheter ablation. Am J Cardiol 1995;76:174–6.

10. Park TH, Eichling JO, Schechtman KB, et al. Risk of radiation induced skin injuries from arrhythmia ablation procedures. Pacing Clin Electrophysiol 1996;19: 1363–9.

11. Rosenthal LS, Beck TJ, Williams J, et al. Acute radiation dermatitis following radiofrequency catheter ablation of atrioventricular nodal reentrant tachycardia. Pacing Clin Electrophysiol 1997;20:1834–9.

12. Mahesh M. Fluoroscopy: patient radiation exposure issues. Radiographics 2001;21:1033–45.

13. Klein LW, Miller DL, Balter S, et al. Occupational health hazards in the interventional laboratory: time for a safer environment. Radiology 2009;250: 538–44.

14. Heidbuchel H, Wittkampf FH, Vano E, et al. Practical ways to reduce radiation dose for patients and staff during device implantations and electrophysiological procedures. Europace 2014;16:946–64.

15. Picano E, Vano E, Rehani MM, et al. The appropriate and justified use of medical radiation in cardiovascular imaging: a position document of the ESC Associations of Cardiovascular Imaging, Percutaneous cardiovascular interventions and electrophysiology. Eur Heart J 2014;35:665–72.

16. Jakobs TF, Becker CR, Ohnesorge B, et al. Multislice helical CT of the heart with retrospective ECG gating: reduction of radiation exposure by ECG-controlled tube current modulation. Eur Radiol 2002;12:1081–6.

17. Ector J, Dragusin O, Adriaenssens B, et al. Obesity is a major determinant of radiation dose in patients undergoing pulmonary vein isolation for atrial fibrillation. J Am Coll Cardiol 2007;50:234–42.

18. Lickfett L, Mahesh M, Vasamreddy C, et al. Radiation exposure during catheter ablation of atrial fibrillation. Circulation 2004;110:3003–10.

19. Venneri L, Rossi F, Botto N, et al. Cancer risk from professional exposure in staff working in cardiac catheterization laboratory: insights from the National Research Council's Biological Effects of Ionizing Radiation VII Report. Am Heart J 2009;157:118–24.

20. Roguin A, Goldstein J, Bar O, et al. Brain and neck tumors among physicians performing interventional procedures. Am J Cardiol 2013;111:1368–72.

21. Agarwal S, Parashar A, Ellis SG, et al. Measures to reduce radiation in a modern cardiac catheterization laboratory. Circ Cardiovasc Interv 2014;7:447–55.

22. Drago F, Silvetti MS, Di Pino A, et al. Exclusion of fluoroscopy during ablation treatment of right

accessory pathway in children. J Cardiovasc Electrophysiol 2002;13:778–82.

23. Smith G, Clark JM. Elimination of fluoroscopy use in a pediatric electrophysiology laboratory utilizing three-dimensional mapping. Pacing Clin Electrophysiol 2007;30:510–8.

24. Tuzcu V. A nonfluoroscopic approach for electrophysiology and catheter ablation procedures using a three-dimensional navigation system. Pacing Clin Electrophysiol 2007;30:519–25.

25. Clark J, Bockoven JR, Lane J, et al. Use of three-dimensional catheter guidance and transesophageal echocardiography to eliminate fluoroscopy in catheter ablation of left-sided accessory pathways. Pacing Clin Electrophysiol 2008;31:283–9.

26. Rossillo A, Indiani S, Bonso A, et al. Novel ICE-guided registration strategy for integration of electroanatomical mapping with three-dimensional CT/MR images to guide catheter ablation of atrial fibrillation. J Cardiovasc Electrophysiol 2009;20:374–8.

27. Singh SM, Heist EK, Donaldson DM, et al. Image integration using intracardiac ultrasound to guide catheter ablation of atrial fibrillation. Heart Rhythm 2008;5:1548–55.

28. Pappone C, Rosanio S, Oreto G, et al. Circumferential radiofrequency ablation of pulmonary vein ostia: a new anatomic approach for curing atrial fibrillation. Circulation 2000;102:2619–28.

29. den Uijl DW, Tops LF, Tolosana JM, et al. Real-time integration of intracardiac echocardiography and multislice computed tomography to guide radiofrequency catheter ablation for atrial fibrillation. Heart Rhythm 2008;5:1403–10.

30. Pratola C, Baldo E, Artale P, et al. Different image integration modalities to guide AF ablation: impact on procedural and fluoroscopy times. Pacing Clin Electrophysiol 2011;34:422–30.

31. Hsu JC, Badhwar N, Gerstenfeld EP, et al. Randomized trial of conventional transseptal needle versus radiofrequency energy needle puncture for left atrial access (the TRAVERSE-LA study). J Am Heart Assoc 2013;2:e000428.

32. Weaver JC. Electroporation: a general phenomenon for manipulating cells and tissues. J Cell Biochem 1993;51:426–35.

33. Whittaker P, Zheng S, Patterson MJ, et al. Histologic signatures of thermal injury: applications in transmyocardial laser revascularization and radiofrequency ablation. Lasers Surg Med 2000;27:305–18.

34. Arana-Rueda E, Pedrote A, Frutos-Lopez M, et al. Electroanatomical mapping of the esophagus in circumferential pulmonary vein isolation. Rev Esp Cardiol 2009;62:1189–92.

35. Huo Y, Christoph M, Forkmann M, et al. Reduction of radiation exposure during atrial fibrillation ablation using a novel fluoroscopy image integrated 3-dimensional electroanatomic mapping system: a

prospective, randomized, single-blind, and controlled study. Heart Rhythm 2015;12:1945–55.

36. Sommer P, Rolf S, Piorkowski C, et al. Nonfluoroscopic catheter visualization in atrial fibrillation ablation: experience from 375 consecutive procedures. Circ Arrhythm Electrophysiol 2014;7:869–74.

37. Sommer P, Bertagnolli L, Kircher S, et al. Safety profile of near-zero fluoroscopy atrial fibrillation ablation with non-fluoroscopic catheter visualization: experience from 1000 consecutive procedures. Europace 2018;20:1952–8.

38. Reddy VY, Morales G, Ahmed H, et al. Catheter ablation of atrial fibrillation without the use of fluoroscopy. Heart Rhythm 2010;7:1644–53.

39. Bulava A, Hanis J, Eisenberger M. Catheter ablation of atrial fibrillation using zero-fluoroscopy technique: a randomized trial. Pacing Clin Electrophysiol 2015; 38:797–806.

40. Liu X, Palmer J. Outcomes of 200 consecutive, fluoroless atrial fibrillation ablations using a new technique. Pacing Clin Electrophysiol 2018;41:1404–11.

41. Sanchez JM, Yanics MA, Wilson P, et al. Fluoroless catheter ablation in adults: a single center experience. J Interv Card Electrophysiol 2016;45:199–207.

42. Percell J, Sharpe E, Percell R. SANS FLUORO (SAy No Series to FLUOROscopy): A First- Year Experience. J Innovations in Cardiac Rhythm Management 2016;7:2529–34.

43. Razminia M, Willoughby MC, Demo H, et al. Fluoroless catheter ablation of cardiac arrhythmias: a 5-year experience. Pacing Clin Electrophysiol 2017; 40:425–33.

Current Status of Esophageal Protection

Rahul Bhardwaj, MD[a], Jacob S. Koruth, MD[b], Vivek Y. Reddy, MD[b],*

KEYWORDS

• Atrial fibrillation • Catheter ablation • Pulmonary vein isolation • Esophagus • Esophageal deviation

KEY POINTS

• Atrial fibrillation ablation can cause thermal injury to the esophagus owing to the proximity of the posterior left atrium to the esophagus.
• The most devastating injury is atrioesophageal fistula, which is almost always fatal.
• Early detection of endoluminal esophageal temperature changes using esophageal temperature probes can decrease the risk of extensive injury.
• Mechanical esophageal deviation can be accomplished with a variety of tools, including off-the-shelf chest tube or dedicated instruments. The extent of esophageal displacement from the site of ablation affects the degree of esophageal temperature elevation.
• Techniques, such as a low irrigation rate, high-power short duration, and using ablation indices to guide radiofrequency ablation may decrease the risk of esophageal injury. Using time-to-isolation to decrease the amount of cryoballoon lesions can also decrease risk to the esophagus.

INTRODUCTION

Catheter ablation is an effective and increasingly common procedure used for the treatment of symptomatic atrial fibrillation (AF). Pulmonary vein isolation (PVI), which includes ablation of the posterior left atrium (LA), is established as an integral component of AF catheter ablation. Damage to the esophagus can occur from the creation of lesions with both radiofrequency (RF) and cryothermy energy in the posterior LA owing to its proximity of the anterior aspect of the esophagus. Thermal ablation lesions can result in collateral damage to surrounding structures such as the esophagus, causing necrosis of esophageal tissue as well as injury to the esophageal blood vessels and nerves.[1]

The most devastating esophageal complication of AF ablation is an atrioesophageal fistula (AEF), which was first described in endocardial surgical RF ablation by Gillinov and colleagues[2] in 2001, and in percutaneous RF catheter ablation by Scanavacca and colleagues[3] and Pappone and colleagues[4] in 2004. AEF has a mortality rate estimated to be 75% and is associated with sepsis and air embolus.[5] The true incidence of esophageal perforation and AEF is not fully appreciated, but is thought to be approximately 0.05% to 0.15%.[6]

Less catastrophic thermal injury to the esophagus occurs relatively more frequently, including mucosal erythema, erosions, and ulceration, as well as esophageal dysmotility caused by damage to the esophageal nerve plexus and vascular structures.[7–9] Knopp and colleagues[8] reported a high rate of pathologic gastrointestinal findings their series of 425 patients who underwent left atrial catheter ablation and follow-up endoscopy after the procedure, including esophageal erythema (21%), gastroparesis (17%), and thermal esophageal lesions (11%). In a pooled analysis, Ha and colleagues[10] found that the incidence of any lesion was 11% and of ulcerated lesions 5% as detected by endoscopy. The majority of erythematous lesions resolve within 2 weeks and

[a] Loma Linda University, 11234 Anderson Street, Room 4404, Loma Linda, CA 92354, USA; [b] Mount Sinai School of Medicine, 1 Gustave L. Levy Place, Suite 1030, New York, NY 10029, USA
* Corresponding author.
E-mail address: Vivek.reddy@mountsinai.org

Card Electrophysiol Clin 12 (2020) 247–257
https://doi.org/10.1016/j.ccep.2020.03.001

1877-9182/20/© 2020 Elsevier Inc. All rights reserved.

ulcerations resolve between 4 and 5 weeks with conservative management.[11]

The burden of esophageal injury is likely underestimated owing to underidentification and reporting of AEF and infrequent routine assessment of esophageal motility after catheter ablation. Furthermore, studying esophageal injury is also made difficult because of the heterogeneity in ablation techniques, power and time settings, and technologies used in addition to patient variability. An understanding and appreciation of esophageal collateral injury has increased in conjunction with greater attention on the role of the posterior LA in the role of AF pathogenesis. The purpose of this article was to review strategies that have been used to understand and mitigate the risk of esophageal injury in AF ablation.

PREDICTING RISK OF ESOPHAGEAL INJURY

Several variables have been identified as risk factors for esophageal injury. The proximity of the esophagus to the site of ablation and specific patient characteristics such as low weight, older age, and higher CHADSVASC score are associated with higher risk.[12] In addition, procedural factors such as ablation technique with RF catheter ablation versus cryoballoon ablation, the use of contact force (CF), and general anesthesia have also been implicated.

Anatomic Factors

The esophagus is a mobile structure in direct contact with the LA that has a varying relationship to the pulmonary veins. Cury and colleagues[13] reported in a series of 65 patients with and without AF who had computed tomography imaging, the esophagus was in direct contact with the posterior LA in all cases with a mean contact width of 18.9 ± 4.4 mm, and was closer to the left pulmonary veins on average. Although additional anatomic factors beyond physical distance of the site of ablation to the esophagus, such as atrial tissue thickness, connective tissue, and adipose tissue, can affect the heat transfer to the esophagus, the physical location of the esophagus remains an important determinant of risk to the esophagus.[14,15]

Defining esophageal position with respect to the LA and PVs can inform on this risk, but is limited in its usefulness because the esophageal position at the time of ablation may be discordant with preprocedural imaging. Further, the esophagus has been demonstrated to shift dynamically during the ablation procedure. In a study of 57 patients undergoing AF ablation under conscious sedation, Daoud and colleagues[16] compared the relationship of the esophagus to the LA as determined by preprocedure versus intraprocedural imaging. Patients had a computed tomography scan 1 week before the ablation, which was then registered to the electroanatomic mapping system, and then performed imaging in real time with an esophagram using orally ingested barium at the time of the ablation procedure. There was concordance of esophageal position with respect to proximity to right versus left pulmonary veins between the 2 modalities in 87% of patients. The investigators noted a significant variation in esophageal position by more than 50% of its diameter during the ablation procedure in 85% of patients.[16] Goode and colleagues[17] also have reported the movement of the esophagus during AF in a series of 51 patients. AF ablation in this series was performed under conscious sedation, and the esophagus was monitored with digital cinefluoroscopic imaging after ingestion of barium paste. The esophagus was observed to move 2 cm or more in 67% of patients, and 4 cm or more in 4% of patients. Periprocedural esophageal movement may not be present in patients undergoing ablation with general anesthesia because peristalsis is disrupted. Predicting the likelihood of esophageal movement could give greater value to esophageal location observed on preprocedure imaging. Yamashita and colleagues[18] have described using the gap between the esophagus between the LA and the vertebral body to predict the likelihood of esophageal movement. Fifty patients undergoing 190 MRI scans were studied with respect to esophageal position and the left atrial–vertebral gap. In this series, 32% of patients were observed to have esophageal movement of more than 10 mm. In their analysis, a left atrial–vertebral gap of 4.5 mm or less was predictive of the esophagus not moving. Thus, although observational studies have found a short distance between the esophagus and LA is associated with a higher risk of esophageal injury, there is evidence to suggest that using preprocedure imaging alone to guide ablation with respect to the esophagus has limitations.[17–20]

Procedural Characteristics

The impact of ablation strategy on esophageal injury risk is important; the goal of creating bigger, contiguous, and more durable lesions is often at odds with minimizing collateral damage. Esophageal injury, including AEF, have been observed with different percutaneous catheter ablation modalities, including RF catheter ablation, cryoballoon ablation, and high-intensity focused ultrasound therapy.[21–24] With respect to RF compared with cryoablation, the mechanism of tissue injury differs significantly but the risk of damage to surrounding structures is shared. The mechanism of RF ablation is resistive heating of myocardial tissue in contact with the catheter, and radial spread of energy with conductive heating that results in denaturation of proteins, including collagen.[25] Cryothermy results in well-circumscribed lesions caused by freezing and thawing, followed by necrosis that typically leaves structural elements intact.[26] Animal studies comparing the modalities on esophageal tissue demonstrated a significant decrease in esophageal tensile strength with RF ablation compared with cryoablation.[27] As such, it was believed that the risk of esophageal injury was significantly less with cryoablation compared with RF ablation. However, cryoballoon AF ablation has been associated with several instances of AEF. Ablation of the left inferior pulmonary vein was observed to be the most frequent injury associated with this complication, which is explained by the relative proximity of the vein to the esophagus.[28] Less severe esophageal damage including thermal lesions and ulcerations, as well as injury to the esophageal nerve plexus, resulting in dysmotility has been described with the second-generation cryoballoon catheter.[29,30] Metzner and colleagues[29] performed a study in 50 patients undergoing AF ablation with the second-generation cryoballoon catheter (Arctic Front Advance, Medtronic, Minneapolis, MN) followed by esophagogastroduodenoscopy (EGD) at 2 ± 1 days after ablation. They found thermal lesions in 2% and esophageal thermal ulceration in 10% of patients. Miyazaki and colleagues[30] in a larger series of 104 patients undergoing ablation with the second-generation cryoballoon catheter followed by esophagogastroscopy reported gastric hypomotility to be present in 17.3% of patients, and esophageal lesions in 8.7% of patients. The proximity of the right inferior pulmonary vein to the esophagus was found to be predictive of gastric hypomotility. A direct comparison of cryoballoon ablation with RF ablation is difficult to accomplish owing to the heterogeneity of RF ablation, but it is clear both modalities can cause esophageal injury.

With the advent of RF ablation catheters capable of assessing CF, operators are able to appreciate the degree of catheter–tissue contact, which has bearing on ablation efficacy. In the TOCCATA study, patients with a low CF (<10 g) experienced recurrence of AF, whereas while those treated with a higher CF (>20 g) were more likely to remain arrhythmia free.[31] The TactiCath Contact Force Ablation Catheter Study for Atrial Fibrillation (TOCCASTAR) study reported that

patients who had optimal CF, which was defined as 90% or more of lesions with 10 g or more CF, were much more likely to have long-term freedom from arrhythmia (75.9% vs 58.1%; P = .018).[32] The overall safety of these catheters is well-established, but limited data exist on the true relationship between CF catheters and relative risk of esophageal injury. An animal study using a canine model demonstrated that at a fixed power and duration, RF energy delivered with a higher CF was associated with higher endoluminal esophageal temperature, a greater frequency of esophageal ulcer development, and larger ulcer size.[33] In a retrospective analysis of the Manufacturer and User Facility Device Experience (MAUDE) database, investigators found a higher incidence of AEF in patients undergoing RF ablation with CF catheters compared those with non-CF catheters (5.4% vs 0.9%; P<.0001). This study is limited in that ablation parameters such as power, time, and duration were referred to. Further, the study is limited in that it is a retrospective analysis of an infrequently recognized and reported procedural complication.[34] Zhang and colleagues[35] conducted the Restricted Contact Force Reduces Esophageal Injury (RESCUE-AF) clinical trial to further investigate the role of CF and esophageal injury. Eighty-nine patients undergoing PVI with a conscious sedation protocol were randomized to CF catheters with goal of a CF of less than 20 g on the posterior wall or to non-CF catheters. A computed tomography scan was obtained before the procedure, which found that the majority of patients had the esophagus positioned near the left pulmonary veins. Endoscopy was performed before and after the ablation procedure. The investigators found that a CF-guided approach with a target of less than 20 g on the posterior wall results in lower rates of esophageal injury compared with non-CF catheters (0% vs 20%).[35] On balance, the informed use of CF catheters in PVI seems to result in greater efficacy and safety, despite reports of a higher AEF incidence.

Several studies have shown a higher risk of esophageal injury with general anesthesia compared with conscious sedation. In a study of 50 patients undergoing catheter ablation for drug-refractory paroxysmal AF using a PVI and superior vena cava isolation approach, Di Biase and colleagues[36] compared the impact of general anesthesia versus conscious sedation with regard to esophageal injury observed using esophageal capsule endoscopy the day after ablation. All patients in the study had luminal esophageal temperature monitoring, and ablation was halted in response to esophageal temperature elevation to greater than 39°C. Ablation was performed using a non–force-sensing irrigated catheter using 45 W for 20 seconds with a temperature limit of 41°C. The investigators observed a small but significantly higher maximum esophageal temperature in the general anesthesia cohort (40.6 ± 1°C vs 39.6 ± 0.8°C; P<.003). They also observed a significantly longer time to baseline temperature recovery (29 ± 3 seconds vs 18 ± 2 seconds; P<.001) and shorter time to peak temperature (9 ± 7 seconds vs 21 ± 9 seconds; P<.001). Esophageal injury was significantly more common in 12 patients (48%) in the general anesthesia arm compared with 1 patient (4%) in the conscious sedation arm. The increased risk of esophageal injury with general anesthesia may be related to the loss of peristaltic waves and not allowing for patient feedback of pain.[36,37]

Despite the plethora of information on esophageal injury, much remains unknown about the risk for esophageal mucosal and functional injury owing to the lack of routine endoscopic evaluation or motility studies in most clinical trials. Additionally, patient factors such as frailty or prior cardiac surgery have not been systematically studied, so identification of high risk patients that warrant closer follow-up is not defined.

- Risk factors for esophageal injury during AF ablation include patient characteristics and proximity of the esophagus to the LA.
- The esophagus is mobile and may shift between the time of the preprocedure imaging and the time of ablation, or even during the ablation itself.
- All thermal ablation modalities, including RF and cryoablation, confer a risk of esophageal injury.
- CF has been reported to be associated with a higher rate of AEF, but prospective studies have demonstrated greater safety and efficacy.
- General anesthesia increases the risk of esophageal injury compared with conscious sedation.

DECREASING THE RISK OF ESOPHAGEAL INJURY

Strategies to decrease gastrointestinal complications include pharmacologic prophylaxis, close monitoring to facilitate early detection of esophageal temperature changes, esophageal interventions to decrease the risks of thermal injury, or changing the ablation approach on the posterior wall of the LA.

Medical Prophylaxis

The role of gastric acid in the development of esophageal lesions after AF ablation is not well-understood, but small studies have noted a higher incidence of endoscopically diagnosed esophageal changes in patients with reflux-like symptoms.[38] Esophageal lesions may worsen owing to the exposure of acidic gastric juice. As such, the use of proton pump inhibitors may be of benefit in decreasing injury. Evidence for the routine use of proton pump inhibitors is sparse, but is generally recommended for 4 to 6 weeks after catheter ablation because the intervention is low risk and can offer benefit.

Luminal Esophageal Temperature Monitoring

Luminal esophageal temperature monitoring has over the years gained in popularity as an approach to detect esophageal thermal exposure during catheter ablation. Various probes are available on the market that differ in shape, in the type of detection sensors, and in the number of sensors, all factors that affect sensitivity.[39] The goal of esophageal temperature monitoring is early detection of injury so ablation can be halted before permanent damage to the esophagus occurs. Although there are limitations with the available technology, recognition of temperature changes at the time of ablation has been shown to be helpful to decrease serious injury.[40–44] Recently, a sensitive infrared thermography catheter was developed to assess esophageal temperatures continuously during catheter ablation. In a study of 16 patients who underwent AF ablation with this catheter placed in the esophagus and had follow-up endoscopy, it was found that patients who had a temperature of greater than 50°C had thermal lesions.[45]

Esophageal temperature probes have been used with cryoballoon ablation procedures as well as RF ablation procedures. The use of esophageal temperature probes with second-generation cryoballoon catheters was found to be predictive of esophageal lesions detected by endoscopy (hazard ratio, 15.750; P = .011) in a prospective study by Miyazaki and associates of 104 patients.[30] Fürnkranz and colleagues[46] reported similar outcomes in 94 patients undergoing PVI with the second-generation cryoballoon ablation catheter. A strategy of interrupting ablation when esophageal temperature reached 15°C resulted in a significant decrease in esophageal lesions without affecting the rate of acute PVI.[46]

Ablation with esophageal temperature probes may result in interrupting ablation owing to esophageal heating, which may result in an ineffective lesion owing to a lack of transmurality because edema may develop before resuming ablation. However, in studies of patients undergoing repeat AF ablation with temperature monitoring, there was no relationship between temperature alerts and acute or chronic reconnections, which suggests that esophageal temperature monitoring does not negatively affect efficacy outcomes.[47,48]

The 2 main criticisms of esophageal temperature monitoring are that (1) probes may not accurately reflect esophageal risk owing to underestimation of esophageal temperature, and (2) the probe itself could directly result in greater esophageal harm. Indeed, the true value remains uncertain; several studies have shown no significant difference in esophageal injury with the use of esophageal temperature probes.[49,50]

Endoluminal ETPs may not accurately detect esophageal wall heating on the extraluminal surface adjacent to the LA, which was suggested by studies that demonstrated a lack of correlation between delivered power and temperature elevation.[10,51] The lack of temperature elevation may be due to the relative proximity of the thermistor to the site of ablation because the thermistor may be displaced laterally or posteriorly. The underestimation of the true temperature could lead to false reassurance and consequent additional ablation and subsequent injury. The second concern that ETPs cause harm is based on 2 putative mechanisms: the probe could act as an antenna and lead to greater injury and the probe could limit peristaltic movement and restrict lateral shift, which could lead to consequent esophageal injury.[52] This effect was observed with probes with unprotected metallic sensors. Computational models have demonstrated that esophageal injury is not electrical, but rather is related to thermal conduction and thus is unlikely to be due to an antenna effect.

Despite these shortcomings, endoluminal esophageal temperature monitoring has been valuable in informing operators on risk to the esophagus with thermal ablation technologies.

Active esophageal cooling

Actively cooling the esophagus has been explored as an option to decrease thermal injury from thermoablation lesions. There are several approaches to cooling the esophagus, including directly cooling the esophagus with ice water or using a cooled esophageal balloon. Directly injecting ice water into the esophagus was explored by Kuwahara and colleagues[53] in 100 patients undergoing RF catheter ablation for AF. Patients were randomized to have ice water injected into the esophagus if the esophageal temperature was observed to reach

42°C or just have ablation halted. There was no significant difference in the presence of esophageal lesions between the 2 groups, although the severity of esophageal lesions seemed to be less in the cooling group.[53] John and colleagues[54] reported similar findings in a series of 76 patients who had luminal esophageal temperature increase by 0.5°C during catheter ablation and were randomized to control versus active esophageal cooling via injection of 20 mL ice water. All patients had a follow-up EGD after ablation, and there was no significant difference in esophageal outcomes, but ablation was less likely to be acutely successful in the cooling group.[54] Specific technologies have been developed to actively cool the esophagus. A cooled water-irrigated intraesophageal balloon has been tested in a small cohort of patients. Luminal esophageal temperature was observed to be relatively lower during ablation.[55] A dedicated esophageal cooling system (EPSac, RossHart Technologies Inc, Cleveland, OH) has been developed to actively circulate temperature-controlled saline or water in a latex sac placed in the esophagus. In an animal study using the system with irrigant at various temperatures, a lower cooling temperature resulted in a decrease in esophageal thermal injury.[56] Further studies are ongoing and are needed to validate this approach.

Mechanical esophageal deviation

Physically displacing the esophagus from the LA is another approach to reduce esophageal injury during thermal ablation as with RF energy. The proximity of the esophagus to the site of ablation is important; conductive thermal injury is thought to be an important mechanism of how esophageal injury is created. Buch and colleagues[57] described placement of an intrapericardial balloon to create a space between the esophagus and the LA during AF ablation. By placing an 18 mm × 4 cm balloon catheter in the oblique sinus adjacent to the LA, a left atrial ablation could be performed without esophageal heating. Cadaver studies demonstrated the feasibility of moving the esophagus.[58,59] Mechanical displacement of the esophagus, thus has been attempted successfully with a variety of techniques, including the use of transesophageal echocardiogram probes, endoscopes, off-the-shelf stylets, as well as more recently certain dedicated instruments.[60–62]

Koruth and colleagues[63] described the use of an off-the-shelf endotracheal stylet placed within a thoracic chest tube to mechanically displace the esophagus an average of 2.8 ± 1.6 cm to the left and 2.8 ± 1.8 cm to the right. Temperature monitoring using a single thermistor temperature probe was used in all patients, and follow-up endoscopy was performed in all patients. The authors found 63% of patients had esophageal instrumentation-related trauma, and 1 patient had a lesion consistent with thermal injury.[63] In a follow-up study, Palaniswamy and colleagues[64] evaluated the extent of esophageal displacement that could be achieved with the stylet and chest tube technique. Contrast was injected into the esophagus after displacement was performed and the distance from the trailing edge to the site of ablation was measured. Effective deviation of at least 20 mm was achieved in 22.2% of attempts and esophageal temperature elevation was found to be related to the degree of separation. More recently, dedicated systems to displace the esophagus during AF ablation have been developed. Two such devices are the DV8 inflatable balloon retractor (Manual Surgical Sciences, Minneapolis, MN) and the EsoSure preshaped nitinol deviator (Northeast Scientific, Waterbury, CT). The DV8 balloon retractor was described in a study of 200 patients undergoing PVI. The system is inserted into the esophagus under general anesthesia, typically after a transseptal puncture has been performed. Contrast is injected using an insufflator into the system to achieve a pressure of approximately 6 ATM. The balloon takes a fixed C shape, and can be manipulated to move the esophagus away from the target ablation site. After completion of the target vein pair, the balloon can be manipulated and positioned in the contralateral position so that the remaining vein pair can be ablated. The extent of effective displacement with this approach was measured, and found to be significantly greater compared with stylet and chest tube technique. Effective deviation of 20 mm or more was achieved in 35.5% of patients, and 13.8% of patients had a deviation between 0 and 10 mm.[65] As in earlier studies, the extent of deviation achieved correlated with the presence of endoluminal esophageal temperature elevation. In the DEFLECT GUT study, Parikh and colleagues[66] reported on the effect of esophageal displacement using the EsoSure device compared with a propensity matched cohort. The EsoSure device is pliable at room temperature and can be shaped to an extent. After insertion into the esophagus, it becomes more rigid at body temperature. In their study, the esophagus was able to be moved an average of 2.45 ± 0.9 cm, and consequently a temperature increase of greater than 1°C was far less frequently seen (3.0% vs 79.4%; $P<.001$).[66] This approach is primarily used for RF ablation but, can be used for other thermal energy sources such as laser and ultrasound ablation. Further studies are needed to determine its safety across multiple operators and its impact on esophageal injury.

ABLATION MODIFICATIONS

The reduced thickness of the posterior LA has led to several approaches that aim to reduce the extent of delivery of ablative energy when ablating the posterior LA. This approach intuitively made sense, but has evolved over time.

Irrigated Radiofrequency Ablation

One of the more common approaches (that has been popular for several years) has centered around limiting power (to approximately 25 W), RF time, and CF on the posterior wall. This approach has been demonstrated to decrease esophageal injury.[35,37,67] Operators who use luminal esophageal temperature monitoring often use additional regional modifications based on degree of luminal esophageal temperature increase and exact parameters vary widely. The major drawback of this strategy has been that it often impacts lesion transmurality and therefore can result in failure to achieve durable pulmonary vein isolation. These approaches have failed to eradicate the issue of esophageal injury, and in particular that of fistula formation.

More recently, modulation of irrigation flow rates was evaluated as a technique to contain the lesion within the myocardium and prevent it from extending into the adjacent esophagus. Kumar and colleagues[68] evaluated this approach in an animal model and demonstrated that ablation using low-flow irrigation (2 mL/min) created atrial lesions with the larger diameter on the endocardial surface as opposed to the epicardial surface, whereas high-flow irrigation created lesions with the larger diameter along the epicardial surface. These investigators then tested this approach in 326 patients undergoing AF ablation; the first 160 patients underwent ablation with 20 to 25 W at high flow (17 mL/min) with a CF of at least 10 g. The subsequent 166 patients underwent ablation using the low-flow strategy. Acute isolation rates were similar between the 2 groups. The authors concluded that, for thin posterior left atrial tissue, the low-flow strategy created equally effective lesions with the potential for improved safety with regard to esophageal injury.[68]

Another recent approach to RF delivery that aims to create shallow lesions is to use high power for short durations. This strategy has become popular and is based on new insights into how irrigated RF creates lesions on thin tissue. It is being increasingly used in posterior left atrial ablation. With this strategy, RF ablation is performed in a point-by-point fashion, using 45 to 50 W applied for durations of less than 10 seconds. This approach to RF delivery relies on the concept that it favors resistive heating over conductive heating, thereby creating a wide but shallow lesion in contrast with the traditional lower power lesions that have their greatest diameter subendocardially. The experience with this approach continues to grow and early reports seem to be favorable.[69] Along these lines, newer modifications to the irrigated RF tip catheters allow for delivery of very high power (90 W) with short durations (4 seconds). Preclinical evaluation of this approach to RF delivery have demonstrated that these lesions were relatively discoid with more radial spread and less depth than lesions created with 25 to 30 W and a longer duration.[70,71] In a study comparing esophageal outcomes based on postprocedure MRI performed 1 day after catheter ablation between 574 patients undergoing ablation with high power for short duration (50 W for 5 seconds) and 113 patients with a standard approach ($\leq$35 W for 10–30 seconds), Baher and colleagues[72] found that esophageal late gadolinium enhancement patterns were similar (64.8% vs 57.5%). Consistent with other studies, procedures with high power for short duration were shorter (149 $\pm$ 65 minutes vs 251 $\pm$ 101 minutes; $P<.001$) and outcomes were similar at 2.5 years of follow-up (42% vs 41%; $P = .571$).[72] Other approaches that have been popularized recently are the use of ablation indices. These indices have been developed to better estimate the lesion size with CF sensing catheters and include proprietary calculations specific to ablation catheters and such as Lesion Size Index and Ablation Index. These approaches have helped to standardize RF delivery per ablation and have been shown to have increased efficacy of AF ablation.[73–75] Studies on esophageal outcomes with a prespecified Ablation Index have also been performed. In 1 study of 211 patient who had EGD performed 1 to 3 days after RF ablation performed at 25 W with a target Ablation Index of 300 to 350 on the posterior wall, the incidence of esophageal lesions detected by endoscopy was 14%.[76] However, in another study of 85 patients that had EGD performed 9 $\pm$ 4 days after ablation at 35 W with a target Ablation Index of 400 (or 300 if the esophageal temperature exceeded 38.5°C), esophageal lesions were observed in only 1 patient (1.2%).[77] Currently, further studies evaluating high power for short duration are on going and will likely result in wider adoption of this approach to limit esophageal injury. The exact definition of high power for short duration seems to vary widely between operators and some modify their delivery to achieve target indices and consensus as to which

approach is best remains to be achieved. In fact, these authors believe that although high power for short duration is attractive conceptually, the wide variation in use of power and time may results in esophageal injury as well.

Cryoablation

Catheter ablation with the cryoballoon, although less likely to result in esophageal injury, is less complex in how it is delivered with respect to limiting esophageal injury. Given that the risk of severe esophageal injury remains with this source, many operators modulate delivery based on luminal esophageal temperature response or use empiric strategies aimed at reducing overall exposure of the esophagus to cryoenergy. Time to isolation (TTI) is a parameter that has been shown to be a predictor of lesion durability and is used to determine the need for additional lesions. This approach has been shown to improve efficacy of cryoballoon PVI.[78,79] Recently, Cordes and colleagues[80] have shown that using TTI-guided cryoballoon ablation can decrease esophageal injury. In 70 patients randomized to TTI-guided ablation or a conventional 2-freeze approach who all underwent EGD after the ablation, patients who had a TTI-guided approach did not have any esophageal lesions, whereas 9% of patients undergoing conventional ablation had thermal lesions.[80] Other approaches involve, interrupting cryoablation if luminal esophageal temperatures decrease to less than a certain level and the use of techniques that optimize positioning.

SUMMARY

The current status of esophageal protection strategies remains widely variable. However, certain specific advances such as the use of high-power short duration RF applications, low-flow irrigation during RF, and the use of mechanical deviation are becoming increasingly popular and their impact on esophageal injury (in particular fistula formation), although encouraging, remains to be assessed comprehensively. Importantly, the recent description of pulsed field ablation for AF ablation seems to be very promising. From the perspective of esophageal safety, it is our hope that if this approach to posterior LA ablation is proven to be also efficacious, then we may finally have in our hands an ability to eradicate esophageal injury risk during AF ablation.[81–83]

DISCLOSURE

Dr V.Y. Reddy: Manual Surgical Sciences and Circa Scientific. Drs R. Bhardwaj and J.S. Koruth have nothing to disclose.

REFERENCES

1. Calkins H, Hindricks G, Cappato R, et al. 2017 HRS/EHRA/ECAS/APHRS/SOLAECE expert consensus statement on catheter and surgical ablation of atrial fibrillation. Europace 2018;20:e1–160.
2. Gillinov AM, Pettersson G, Rice TW, et al. Esophageal injury during radiofrequency ablation for atrial fibrillation. J Thorac Cardiovasc Surg 2001;122:1239–40.
3. Scanavacca MI, D'ávila A, Parga J, et al. Left atrial esophageal fistula following radiofrequency catheter ablation of atrial fibrillation. J Cardiovasc Electrophysiol 2004;15:960–2.
4. Pappone C, Oral H, Santinelli V, et al. Atrio-esophageal fistula as a complication of percutaneous transcatheter ablation of atrial fibrillation. Circulation 2004;109:2724–6.
5. Kadaria D, Mountjoy LJ, Priaulx AB, et al. Atrioesophageal fistula: a case series and literature review. Am J Case Rep 2017;18:847–54.
6. Ghia KK, Chugh A, Good E, et al. A nationwide survey on the prevalence of atrioesophageal fistula after left atrial radiofrequency catheter ablation. J Interv Card Electrophysiol 2009;24:33–6.
7. Halm U, Gaspar T, Zachäus M, et al. Thermal esophageal lesions after radiofrequency catheter ablation of left atrial arrhythmias. Am J Gastroenterol 2010;105:551–6.
8. Knopp H, Halm U, Lamberts R, et al. Incidental and ablation-induced findings during upper gastrointestinal endoscopy in patients after ablation of atrial fibrillation: a retrospective study of 425 patients. Heart Rhythm 2014;11:574–8.
9. Lakkireddy D, Reddy YM, Atkins D, et al. Effect of atrial fibrillation ablation on gastric motility: the atrial fibrillation gut study. Circ Arrhythm Electrophysiol 2015;8:531–6.
10. Ha FJ, Han HC, Sanders P, et al. Prevalence and prevention of oesophageal injury during atrial fibrillation ablation: a systematic review and meta-analysis. Europace 2019;21:80–90.
11. Yarlagadda B, Deneke T, Turagam M, et al. Temporal relationships between esophageal injury type and progression in patients undergoing atrial fibrillation catheter ablation. Heart Rhythm 2019;16:204–12.
12. Kim YG, Shim J, Kim DH, et al. Characteristics of atrial fibrillation patients suffering atrioesophageal fistula after radiofrequency catheter ablation. J Cardiovasc Electrophysiol 2018;29:1343–51.
13. Cury RC, Abbara S, Schmidt S, et al. Relationship of the esophagus and aorta to the left atrium and pulmonary veins: implications for catheter ablation of atrial fibrillation. Heart Rhythm 2005;2:1317–23.
14. Ito M, Yamabe H, Koyama J, et al. Analysis for the primary predictive factor for the incidence of esophageal injury after ablation of atrial fibrillation. J Cardiol 2018;72:480–7.
15. Sánchez-Quintana D, Cabrera JA, Climent V, et al. Anatomic relations between the esophagus and left atrium and relevance for ablation of atrial fibrillation. Circulation 2005;112:1400–5.
16. Daoud EG, Hummel JD, Houmsse M, et al. Comparison of computed tomography imaging with intraprocedural contrast esophagram: implications for catheter ablation of atrial fibrillation. Heart Rhythm 2005;5:975–80.
17. Goode E, Lemola K, Han J, et al. Movement of the esophagus during left atrial catheter ablation for atrial fibrillation. J Am Coll Cardiol 2005;46:2107–10.
18. Kobza R, Schoenenberger AW, Erne P. Esophagus imaging for catheter ablation of atrial fibrillation: comparison of two methods with showing of esophageal movement. J Interv Card Electrophysiol 2009;26:159–64.
19. Starek Z, Lehar F, Jez J, et al. Three-dimensional rotational angiography of the left atrium and the oesophagus: the short-term mobility of the oesophagus and the stability of the fused three-dimensional model of the left atrium and the oesophagus during catheter ablation for atrial fibrillation. Europace 2017;19:1310–6.
20. Yamashita K, Quang C, Schroeder JD, et al. Distance between the left atrium and the vertebral body is predictive of esophageal movement in serial MR imaging. J Interv Card Electrophysiol 2018;52:149–56.
21. Barbhaiya CR, Kumar S, Guo Y, et al. Global survey of esophageal and gastric injury in atrial fibrillation ablation: characteristics and outcomes of esophageal perforation and fistula. JACC Clin Electrophysiol 2016;2:143–50.
22. Chavez P, Messerli FH, Casso Dominguez A, et al. Atrioesophageal fistula following ablation procedures for atrial fibrillation: systematic review of case reports. Open Heart 2015;2:e000257.
23. Stöckigt F, Schrickel JW, Andrié R, et al. Atrioesophageal fistula after cryoballoon pulmonary vein isolation. J Cardiovasc Electrophysiol 2012;23:1254–7.
24. Neven K, Schmidt B, Metzner A, et al. Fatal end of a safety algorithm for pulmonary vein isolation with use of high-intensity focused ultrasound. Circ Arrhythm Electrophysiol 2010;3:260–5.
25. Kok L, Everett T, Akar J, et al. Effect of heating on pulmonary veins: how to avoid pulmonary vein stenosis. J Cardiovasc Electrophysiol 2003;14:250–4.
26. Lustgarten D, Keane D, Ruskin J. Cryothermal ablation: mechanism of tissue injury and current experience in the treatment of tachyarrhythmias. Prog Cardiovasc Dis 1999;41:481–98.
27. Evonich RF III, Nori DM, Haines DE. A randomized trial comparing effects of radiofrequency and

cryoablation on the structural integrity of esophageal tissue. J Interv Card Electrophysiol 2007;19:77–83.

28. John RM, Kapur S, Ellenbogen KA, et al. Atrioesophageal fistula formation with cryo-balloon ablation is most commonly related to the left inferior pulmonary vein. Heart Rhythm 2017;14:184–9.

29. Metzner A, Burchard A, Wohlmuth P, et al. Increased incidence of esophageal thermal lesions using the second-generation 28-mm cryoballoon. Circ Arrhythm Electrophysiol 2013;6:769–75.

30. Miyazaki S, Nakamura H, Taniguchi H, et al. Gastric hypomotility after second-generation cryoballoon ablation—unrecognized silent nerve injury after cryoballoon ablation. Heart Rhythm 2017;14:670–7.

31. Reddy VY, Shah D, Kautzner J, et al. The relationship between contact force and clinical outcome during radiofrequency catheter ablation of atrial fibrillation in the TOCCATA study. Heart Rhythm 2012;9:1789–95.

32. Reddy VY, Dukkipati SR, Neuzil P, et al. Randomized, controlled trial of the safety and effectiveness of a contact force–sensing irrigated catheter for ablation of paroxysmal atrial fibrillation. Circulation 2015;132:907–15.

33. Nakagawa H, Ikeda A, Shah D, et al. Role of contact force in esophageal injury during left atrial radiofrequency ablation. Heart Rhythm 2008;5:s308–33.

34. Black-Maier E, Pokorney SD, Barnett AS, et al. Risk of atrioesophageal fistula formation with contact force-sensing catheters. Heart Rhythm 2017;14:1328–33.

35. Zhang X, Kuang X, Gao X, et al. RESCUE-AF in patients undergoing atrial fibrillation ablation. Circ Arrhythm Electrophysiol 2019;12:e007044.

36. Di Biase L, Saenz LC, Burkhardt DJ, et al. Esophageal capsule endoscopy after radiofrequency catheter ablation for atrial fibrillation: documented higher risk of luminal esophageal damage with general anesthesia as compared with conscious sedation. Circ Arrhythm Electrophysiol 2009;2:108–12.

37. Martinek M, Bencsik G, Aichinger J, et al. Esophageal damage during radiofrequency ablation of atrial fibrillation: impact of energy settings, lesion sets, and esophageal visualization. J Cardiovasc Electrophysiol 2009;20:726–33.

38. Schmidt M, Nolker G, Marschang H, et al. Incidence of oesophageal wall injury post-pulmonary vein antrum isolation for treatment of patients with atrial fibrillation. Europace 2008;10:205–9.

39. Turagam MK, Miller S, Sharma SP, et al. Differences in transient thermal response of commercial esophageal temperature probes. JACC Clin Electrophysiol 2019;5:1280–8.

40. Singh SM, d'Avila A, Doshi SK, et al. Esophageal injury and temperature monitoring during atrial fibrillation ablation. Circ Arrhythm Electrophysiol 2008;1:162–8.

41. Kuwahara T, Takahashi A, Kobori A, et al. Safe and effective ablation of atrial fibrillation: importance of esophageal temperature monitoring to avoid periesophageal nerve injury as a complication of pulmonary vein isolation. J Cardiovasc Electrophysiol 2008;20:1–6.

42. Kiuchi K, Okajima K, Shimane A, et al. Impact of esophageal temperature monitoring guided atrial fibrillation ablation on preventing asymptomatic excessive transmural injury. J Arrhythm 2015;32:36–41.

43. Ito M, Yamabe H, Kanazawa H, et al. Analysis of the usefulness of esophageal temperature monitoring for the prevention of esophageal injury after catheter ablation of atrial fibrillation: its relation to the distance between the esophagus and left atrium. Circulation 2018;138. Suppl1 abstract 12488.

44. Sause A, Tutdibi O, Pomsel K, et al. Limiting esophageal temperature in radiofrequency ablation of left atrial tachyarrhythmias results in low incidence of thermal esophageal lesions. BMC Cardiovasc Disorders 2010;10:52.

45. Daly MG, Melton I, Roper G, et al. High-resolution infrared thermography of esophageal temperature during radiofrequency ablation of atrial fibrillation. Circ Arrhythm Electrophysiol 2018;11:e005667.

46. Fürnkranz A, Bordignon S, Böhmig M, et al. Reduced incidence of esophageal lesions by luminal esophageal temperature-guided second-generation cryoballoon ablation. Heart Rhythm 2015;12:268–74.

47. Leo M, Pedersen MF, Rajappan K, et al. Premature termination of radiofrequency delivery during pulmonary vein isolation due to oesophageal temperature alerts: impact on acute and chronic pulmonary vein reconnection. Europace 2017;19:954–60.

48. Kimura T, Nishiyama N, Negashi M, et al. The durability of atrial fibrillation ablation using an oesophageal temperature cut-off of 38 °C. Heart Lung Circ 2019;28:1050–8.

49. Gianni C, Atoui M, Mohanty S, et al. Difference in thermodynamics between two types of esophageal temperature probes: insights from an experimental study. Heart Rhythm 2016;13:2195–200.

50. Kuwahara T, Takahashi A, Takahashi Y, et al. Incidences of esophageal injury during esophageal temperature monitoring: a comparative study of a multi-thermocouple temperature probe and a deflectable temperature probe in atrial fibrillation ablation. J Interv Card Electrophysiol 2014;39:251–7.

51. Cummings JE, Barrett CD, Litwak KN, et al. Esophageal luminal temperature measurement underestimates esophageal tissue temperature during radiofrequency ablation within the canine left atrium: comparison between 8 mm tip and open irrigation

catheters. J Cardiovasc Electrophysiol 2008;19:
641–4.

52. Nguyen DT, Barham W, Zheng L, et al. Effect of radiofrequency energy delivery in proximity to metallic medical device components. Heart Rhythm 2015; 12:2162–9.

53. Kuwahara T, Takahashi A, Okubo K, et al. Oesophageal cooling with ice water does not reduce the incidence of oesophageal lesions complicating catheter ablation of atrial fibrillation: randomized controlled study. Europace 2014;16:834–9.

54. John J, Garg L, Orosey M, et al. The effect of esophageal cooling on esophageal injury during radiofrequency catheter ablation of atrial fibrillation. J Interv Card Electrophysiol 2019;1–8. [Epub ahead of print].

55. Tsuchiya T, Ashikaga K, Nakagawa S, et al. Atrial fibrillation ablation with esophageal cooling with a cooled water-irrigated intraesophageal balloon: a pilot study. J Cardiovasc Electrophysiol 2007;18: 145–50.

56. Arruda MS, Armaganijan L, Di Biase L, et al. Feasibility and safety of using an esophageal protective system to eliminate esophageal thermal injury: implications on atrial-esophageal fistula following AF ablation. J Cardiovasc Electrophysiol 2009;20: 1272–8.

57. Buch E, Nakahara S, Shivkumar K. Intra-pericardial balloon retraction of the left atrium: a novel method to prevent esophageal injury during catheter ablation. Heart Rhythm 2008;5:1473–5.

58. Krishnan SC, Salazar M, Narula N. Anatomical basis for the mobility of the esophagus: implications for catheter ablation of atrial fibrillation. Indian Pacing Electrophysiol J 2008;8:66–8.

59. Marar D, Muthusamy V, Krishnan SC. Avoiding oesophageal injury during cardiac ablation: insights gained from mediastinal anatomy. Europace 2018; 20:266–71.

60. Herweg B, Johnson N, Postler G, et al. Mechanical esophageal deflection during ablation of atrial fibrillation. Pacing Clin Electrophysiol 2006;29:957–61.

61. Mateós JC, Mateós E, Peña S, et al. Simplified method for esophagus protection during radiofrequency catheter ablation of atrial fibrillation - prospective study of 704 cases. Rev Bras Cir Cardiovasc 2015;30(2):139–47.

62. Chugh A, Rubenstein J, Good E, et al. Mechanical displacement of the esophagus in patients undergoing left atrial ablation of atrial fibrillation. Heart Rhythm 2009;6:319–22.

63. Koruth JS, Reddy VY, Miller MA, et al. Mechanical esophageal displacement during catheter ablation for atrial fibrillation. J Cardiovasc Electrophysiol 2011;23:147–54.

64. Palaniswamy C, Koruth JS, Mittnacht AJ, et al. The extent of mechanical esophageal deviation to avoid

esophageal heating during catheter ablation of atrial fibrillation. JACC Clin Electrophysiol 2017;3: 1146–54.

65. Bhardwaj R, Naniwadekar A, Whang W, et al. Esophageal deviation during atrial fibrillation ablation: clinical experience with a dedicated esophageal balloon retractor. JACC Clin Electrophysiol 2018;4: 1020–30.

66. Parikh V, Swarup V, Hantla J, et al. Feasibility, safety, and efficacy of a novel preshaped nitinol esophageal deviator to successfully deflect the esophagus and ablate left atrium without esophageal temperature rise during atrial fibrillation ablation: the DEFLECT GUT study. Heart Rhythm 2018;15: 1321–7.

67. Chelu MG, Morris AK, Kholmovski EG, et al. Durable lesion formation while avoiding esophageal injury during ablation of atrial fibrillation: lessons learned from late gadolinium MR imaging. J Cardiovasc Electrophysiol 2018;29:385–92.

68. Kumar S, Romero J, Stevenson WG, et al. Impact of lowering irrigation flow rate on atrial lesion formation in thin atrial tissue. JACC Clin Electrophysiol 2017;3: 1114–25.

69. Winkle RA, Mohant S, Patrawala RA, et al. Low complication rates using high power (45–50 W) for short duration for atrial fibrillation ablations. Heart Rhythm 2019;16:165–9.

70. Leshem E, Zilberman I, Tschabrunn CM, et al. High-power and short-duration ablation for pulmonary vein isolation. JACC Clin Electrophysiol 2018;4: 467–79.

71. Reddy VY, Grimaldi M, De Potter T, et al. Pulmonary vein isolation with very high power, short duration, temperature-controlled lesions. JACC Clin Electrophysiol 2019;5:778–86.

72. Baher A, Kheirkhakha M, Rechenmacher SJ, et al. High-power radiofrequency catheter ablation of atrial fibrillation: using late gadolinium enhancement magnetic resonance imaging as a novel index of esophageal injury. JACC Clin Electrophysiol 2018; 4:1583–94.

73. Neuzil P, Kuck KH, Nakagawa H, et al. Lesion size index for prediction of reconnection risk following RF ablation for PVI [abstract]. Heart Rhythm Society, Boston, May 9-12, 2012. Heart Rhythm 2012;9(5 Suppl 1):S492. Abstract MP04-03.

74. Sundaram S, Choe W, Jordan JR, et al. Two year, single center clinical outcome after catheter ablation for paroxysmal atrial fibrillation guided by lesion index. J Atr Fibrillation 2018;11:1760.

75. Phlips T, Taghji P, El Haddad M, et al. Improving procedural and one-year outcome after contact force-guided pulmonary vein isolation: the role of interlesion distance, ablation index, and contact force variability in the 'CLOSE'-protocol. Europace 2018;20: f419-f427.

76. Halbfass P, Berkovitz A, Pavlov B, et al. Incidence of acute thermal esophageal injury after atrial fibrillation ablation guided by prespecified ablation index. J Cardiovasc Electrophysiol 2019;30:2256–61.

77. Wolf M, Haddad ME, De Wilde V, et al. Endoscopic evaluation of the esophagus after catheter ablation of atrial fibrillation using contiguous and optimized radiofrequency applications. Heart Rhythm 2019; 16:1013–20.

78. Reissmann B, Wissner E, Deiss S, et al. First insights into cryoballoon-based pulmonary vein isolation taking the individual time-to-isolation into account. Europace 2017;19:1676–80.

79. Julian Chun KR, Stich M, Fürnkranz A, et al. Individualized cryoballoon energy pulmonary vein isolation guided by real-time pulmonary vein recordings, the randomized ICE-T trial. Heart Rhythm 2017;14: 495–500.

80. Cordes F, Ellermann C, Dechering DG, et al. Time-to-isolation-guided cryoballoon ablation reduces oesophageal and mediastinal alterations detected by endoscopic ultrasound: results of the MADE-PVI trial. Europace 2019;21:1325–33.

81. Reddy VY, Koruth JS, Jais P, et al. Ablation of atrial fibrillation with pulsed electric fields: an ultra-rapid, tissue-selective modality for cardiac ablation. JACC Clin Electrophysiol 2018;4(8):987–95.

82. Reddy VY, Neuzil P, Koruth JS, et al. Pulsed field ablation for pulmonary vein isolation in atrial fibrillation. J Am Coll Cardiol 2019;74(3):315–26.

83. Neven K, van Es R, van Driel V, et al. Acute and long-term effects of full-power electroporation ablation directly onto the porcine esophagus. Circ Arrhythm Electrophysiol 2017;10:e004672.

Discontinuing Anticoagulation After Catheter Ablation of Atrial Fibrillation

Naga Venkata K. Pothineni, MD, David S. Frankel, MD*

KEYWORDS

- Atrial fibrillation • Anticoagulation • Catheter ablation • Oral anticoagulants
- Direct-acting oral anticoagulants

KEY POINTS

- Atrial fibrillation is a leading cause of ischemic stroke.
- Stroke risk can be reduced with oral anticoagulation; however, the accompanying increase in bleeding risk is unavoidable.
- Current guidelines recommend that decisions regarding anticoagulation after ablation be based solely on preprocedural risk, as defined by established risk scores.
- Whether the absolute risk of stroke is sufficiently reduced by successful catheter ablation such that the benefit in terms of further reduction in strokes with continued oral anticoagulation is outweighed by increased bleeds, remains to be determined.
- Observational data suggest that in appropriately selected patients, oral anticoagulation can be stopped after successful atrial fibrillation ablation without an unacceptably high increase in stroke risk.

INTRODUCTION

Atrial fibrillation (AF) is the most common, sustained cardiac arrhythmia worldwide, with a steadily increasing prevalence. It is estimated that more than 6 million adults in the United States have AF, with the number expected to double by 2050.[1] Ischemic stroke remains the most feared consequence of AF, with more than one-third of all ischemic strokes attributable to AF. Anticoagulation with vitamin K antagonists or direct acting oral anticoagulants (DOACs) is well-established as the standard of care for stroke prevention. However, long-term anticoagulation increases risk of major bleeding, which in turn increases

morbidity and mortality. Clinicians managing patients with AF must balance risks of stroke and bleeding to optimize outcomes for their patients.

Catheter ablation (CA) for AF has steadily improved over the past 2 decades, leading to better rates of arrhythmia control and improved quality of life. The impact of AF ablation on stroke risk remains to be fully defined. Current practice guidelines recommend continuing anticoagulation after ablation, according to the preablation estimated stroke risk as defined by risk scores such as the CHA_2DS_2-VASc,[2] regardless of the perceived success of ablation.[3] However, clinicians frequently encounter patients who would prefer to stop anticoagulation after AF ablation for multiple reasons.

Section of Cardiac Electrophysiology, Division of Cardiovascular Medicine, Perelman School of Medicine at the University of Pennsylvania, 3400 Spruce Street, 9 Founders Pavilion, Philadelphia, PA 19104, USA
* Corresponding author. Hospital of the University of Pennsylvania, 3400 Spruce Street, 9 Founders Pavilion, Philadelphia, PA 19104, USA.
E-mail address: david.frankel@pennmedicine.upenn.edu

Card Electrophysiol Clin 12 (2020) 259–264
https://doi.org/10.1016/j.ccep.2020.02.007
1877-9182/20/© 2020 Elsevier Inc. All rights reserved.

Sophisticated patients often question the applicability of AF stoke risk estimators when they are no longer having AF after ablation. Although randomized trial data are not yet available to guide this decision, deductions can be made from observational data and clinical reasoning. Here, we review the pathophysiologic relationship between AF and ischemic stroke, review the observational data pertaining to anticoagulation discontinuation after CA and describe the authors' current practices in this regard.

PATHOPHYSIOLOGY OF ATRIAL FIBRILLATION AND STROKE

Although epidemiologic associations between AF and ischemic stroke are well-established, the specific mechanistic causes are actively debated. The long-standing, dominant theory is that AF induced stasis in the left atrium results in thrombosis and embolization. However, recent evidence points toward a more complex relationship, involving extensive substrate changes in atrial architecture, termed atrial cardiopathy.[4] This theory argues that atrial fibrosis and dysfunction drive stroke risk, with AF merely an epiphenomenon. This theory is supported by a lack of temporal correlation between AF episodes and cardioembolic events.[5] Further, the CHA_2DS_2-VASc score has been criticized as a predictor of cardiovascular disease burden in general, rather than AF stroke risk in particular. In a large, prospective, registry study from Canada, CHA_2DS_2-VASc potently predicted ischemic stroke among patients without AF.[6] It is possible that the power of the CHA_2DS_2-VASc score could be improved by incorporating physiologic parameters indicative of the extent of atrial cardiopathy. For example, a large meta-analysis of 9 cohort studies including 67,875 patients showed that left atrial size is strongly associated with risk of ischemic stroke.[7] More recent advances in imaging have helped to identify atrial fibrosis as an incremental risk factor for stroke, beyond traditional scoring systems.[8] The impact of successful AF ablation on left atrial size and fibrosis, in addition to reduction in AF burden, could potentially modulate postablation stroke risk.

REAL-WORLD ANTICOAGULATION PRACTICES AFTER ATRIAL FIBRILLATION ABLATION

Current practice guidelines recommend continuing anticoagulation indefinitely after AF ablation, according to stroke risk estimators.[3] However, significant practice variations exist, with each decision driven by an individual patient and provider. In a Canadian survey, 95% of electrophysiologists would discontinue oral anticoagulation (OAC) after successful ablation in a hypothetical patient with a CHADS2 score of 1 or less.[9] In a European survey of electrophysiologists, 16% felt comfortable stopping anticoagulation after successful CA in hypothetical patients with a CHADS2 score of 2 or greater.[10] Increasing comfort with stopping anticoagulation seems to be related to low reported rates of ischemic stroke after AF ablation. Using a large, national, administrative claims database, Noseworthy and colleagues[11] analyzed patterns of OAC use after CA for AF over a 10-year period. In their study of 6886 patients, they reported OAC discontinuation rates of 82% and 62.5% at 12 months for patients with CHA_2DS_2-VASc scores of 0 to 1 and 2 or greater, respectively. The risk of stroke and systemic embolism was higher among patients with CHA_2DS_2-VASc scores of 2 or greater who stopped anticoagulation, compared with similar patients who did not stop anticoagulation. No such increase in risk was observed among patients with CHA_2DS_2-VASc scores of 1 or less. In a recent meta-analysis of 5 studies, Romero and colleagues[12] similarly reported a beneficial effect of continuing OAC in patients with higher risk. In this analysis, the use of anticoagulation beyond the 3-month period after CA was associated with a 59% relative reduction in the risk of thromboembolic events in patients with a CHA_2DS_2-VASc score of 2 or greater. However, there was also a statistically significant increase in the risk of intracranial hemorrhage. In the Danish nationwide registry, Karasoy and colleagues[13] evaluated the risk of thromboembolic and major bleeding events in a cohort of 4050 patients undergoing first-time AF ablation with a mean follow-up of 3.6 years. They found that OAC discontinuation was associated with a 0.6% higher risk of thromboembolism and a 1.8% lower risk of serious bleeding, defined as hospitalization for intracranial bleeding, or bleeding from the respiratory, gastrointestinal, or urinary tract. Recurrent AF and a prior history of stroke were independent predictors of thromboembolic events, although there was no difference in stroke rates based on CHA_2DS_2-VASc score alone.

In a multicenter study, Themistoclakis and colleagues[14] evaluated the safety of stopping anticoagulation 3 to 6 months after successful AF ablation in 2692 patients. Over median of 2 years of follow-up, the incidence of ischemic stroke was only 0.07%. Rates of major hemorrhage were significantly higher among those who continued anticoagulation (2.00% vs 0.04% among those who stopped anticoagulation; $P<.0001$). Other studies have shown that maintenance of sinus rhythm after ablation is the most important predictor of stroke. For example, Nademanee and colleagues[15] reported annual stroke rates of 0.4% among patients taken off anticoagulation after successful ablation, who continued to remain in sinus rhythm. In this study, annual stroke rates in patient who continued warfarin was significantly higher at 2%, pointing toward a relation between postablation AF burden and stroke rates. Riley and colleagues[16] analyzed data from all AF ablations performed at the University of Pennsylvania from 2000 to 2009. In this analysis of 1990 ablations, warfarin was discontinued in more than one-half of patients (52%). There were a total of 16 thromboembolic events (incident rate of 0.2% per patient year). One-half of these thromboembolic events occurred in patients on OAC and the majority had preceding AF recurrence. The incidence of major bleeding was significantly higher in the group of patients that continued OAC (1.4% vs 0.1%; $P<.01$). In this study, postablation strokes were better predicted by AF recurrence than CHADS2 scores. More than one-third of all strokes occurred in patients with a CHADS2 of 0, who would typically be considered low risk.

MONITORING FOR ATRIAL FIBRILLATION RECURRENCE AFTER ABLATION

A wide variety of tools are now available to monitor for AF recurrence after ablation, some of which enable rapid identification of AF with a potential for prompt reinitiation of OAC. These range from smart watches to medical-grade wearable monitors and insertable cardiac monitors (ICM). It stands to reason that the more prolonged the duration of monitoring, the greater the sensitivity for recurrent AF. In a single-center study, ICMs were inserted in 65 patients with mean a CHA_2DS_2-VASc score of 2.8, who remained AF free 3 months after ablation.[17] OAC was stopped in all patients. Over a mean of 32 months of follow-up, AF lasting more than 1 hour was detected in 32% of patients. OAC was restarted in these patients, whereas the remaining 68% remained off OAC. No thromboembolic events occurred in either group. Pulse monitoring is another technique used to detect AF after ablation. Although this technique is free, readily available, and long lasting, it requires active participation by the patient. Regular pulse monitoring at least twice a day and with symptoms is considered essential at our institution and patients are trained to do so.

ATRIAL FIBRILLATION-TRIGGERED ANTICOAGULATION

With their rapid onset of action, DOACs open the potential for anticoagulation as needed for AF recurrence, often termed the pill in the pocket approach. The Rhythm Evaluation for Anticoagulation with Continuous Monitoring (REACT.COM) pilot study evaluated the feasibility of using ICMs to detect episodes of AF and initiate treatment with DOACs, as opposed to continuous anticoagulation while in sinus rhythm.[18] In this multicenter, prospective study, patients with nonvalvular AF and a CHADS2 score of greater than 1 who had no evidence of AF during a 2-month run-in period were included. Any detected AF episode greater than 1 hour triggered use of a DOAC for a 4-week period. If AF again recurred within the following 30 days, the DOAC would be continued indefinitely. If AF did not recur again within the 30 days after AF detection, OAC was stopped and monitoring continued. In this study of 59 patients with more than 1 year of follow-up, ICM-guided anticoagulation strategy led to a 94% decrease in overall time on anticoagulation. There were 3 transient ischemic attacks and no strokes. A large, multicenter, prospective trial of smart phone electrocardiogram-guided anticoagulation, the REACT-AF trial is currently being planned, again examining the pill in the pocket approach of anticoagulation with DOACs in patients with nonvalvular AF.[19]

This pill in the pocket approach also seems to be a promising alternative to continuous anticoagulation after successful CA for AF. Zado and colleagues[20] retrospectively examined this approach in 99 patients after successful ablation. This patient population was carefully selected and were capable of pulse assessment twice daily, had no AF detected during extensive monitoring after AF ablation, a left atrial diameter of less than 5 cm, and no evidence of spontaneous echo contrast noted on intracardiac echocardiography performed during the ablation procedure. All patients were instructed to start DOAC for episodes of AF more than 1 hour or recurrent shorter episodes. When a DOAC was started for recurrent AF episodes, the usual duration of therapy was 2 to 4 weeks. In this study, 18% of patients transitioned to daily DOACs for frequent recurrences of AF. Over mean follow-up 30 ± 14 months, a single transient ischemic attack occurred. With emerging technology that makes AF detection easier, OAC triggered by recurrence becomes more feasible.

ONGOING RANDOMIZED CONTROLLED TRIALS

Two major randomized trials are currently underway examining discontinuation of OAC after AF ablation. The Oral Anticoagulation Therapy Pilot

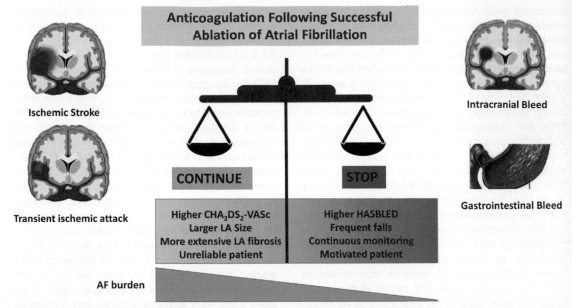

Fig. 1. Factors impacting the decision to continue OAC after AF ablation. A higher stroke risk as defined by traditional risk scores, as well as physiologic markers of atrial cardiopathy, favors continuing anticoagulation. A greater risk of bleeding, as well more extensive monitoring showing no recurrence, favors stopping anticoagulation. If anticoagulation is stopped, the patient must be instructed to perform pulse checks and restart anticoagulation in the event of irregularity. LA, left atrium.

Study (OAT) completed enrollment of 100 patients in October 2019. It included patients with a CHA$_2$-DS$_2$-VASc score of 3 or greater with no evidence of AF recurrence during extended monitoring for 3 months after ablation.[21] Patients were then randomized to stop versus continue OAC. The primary outcome is a composite of thromboembolic and hemorrhagic events during 12-month follow-up. The larger Optimal Anti-Coagulation for Enhanced-Risk Patients Post–Catheter Ablation for Atrial Fibrillation (OCEAN) trial is a randomized, multicenter trial planning to enroll 1572 patients with AF and a CHA$_2$DS$_2$-VASc score of 1 or greater who are free of AF 12 months after ablation.[22] Patients are then randomized to rivaroxaban 15 mg/d or aspirin 75 to 160 mg/d. Brain MRIs are being

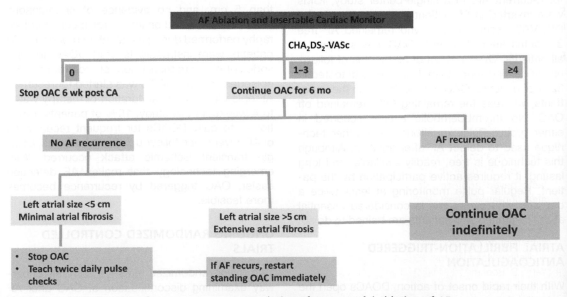

Fig. 2. Proposed algorithm for managing anticoagulation after successful ablation of AF.

performed to assess for asymptomatic cerebral emboli. Given the size and randomized nature of this trial, the potential to impact practice is high.

SUMMARY AND RECOMMENDATIONS

AF is a leading cause of ischemic stroke. Stroke risk can be reduced with OAC; however, the accompanying increase in bleeding risk is unavoidable. Current guidelines recommend that decisions regarding anticoagulation after ablation be based solely on preprocedural risk, as defined by established risk scores. Whether the absolute risk of stroke is sufficiently reduced by successful CA such that the benefit in terms of further reduction in strokes with continued OAC is outweighed by increased bleeds, remains to be determined. Observational data suggest that, in appropriately selected patients, OAC can be stopped after successful AF ablation without an unacceptably high increase in stroke risk. A large randomized trial testing this hypothesis is currently under way. Factors that favor stopping OAC after AF ablation include lower CHA_2DS_2-VASc score, a lesser extent of atrial cardiopathy as defined by atrial size and fibrosis and higher bleeding risk (**Fig. 1**). More extensive monitoring with ICMs, smart devices and frequent pulse checks provide greater sensitivity for recurrence. Whether a strategy of as needed OAC can provide the best of both strategies (adequate protection from stroke with lower risk of bleeding), also remains to be established. The authors' strategy for managing OAC after AF ablation is illustrated in **Fig. 2**.

DISCLOSURE

Supported by the Pennsylvania Steel Company EP Research Fund.

REFERENCES

1. Mozaffarian D, Benjamin EJ, Go AS, et al. Heart disease and stroke statistics: 2015 update: a report from the American Heart Association. Circulation 2015;131:e29–322.
2. Lip GY, Nieuwlaat R, Pisters R, et al. Refining clinical risk stratification for predicting stroke and thromboembolism in atrial fibrillation using a novel risk factor-based approach: the euro heart survey on atrial fibrillation. Chest 2010;137(2):263–72.
3. Calkins H, Hindricks G, Cappato R, et al. 2017 HRS/EHRA/ECAS/APHRS/SOLAECE expert consensus statement on catheter and surgical ablation of atrial fibrillation. Heart Rhythm 2017;14:e275–444.
4. Yaghi S, Boehme AK, Hazan R, et al. Atrial cardiopathy and cryptogenic stroke: a cross-sectional pilot study. J Stroke Cerebrovasc Dis 2016;25(1):110–4.
5. Brambatti M, Connolly SJ, Gold MR, et al. Temporal relationship between subclinical atrial fibrillation and embolic events. Circulation 2014;129(21):2094–9.
6. Mitchell LB, Southern DA, Galbraith D, et al. Prediction of stroke or TIA in patients without atrial fibrillation using CHADS2 and CHA2DS2-VASc scores. Heart 2014;100(19):1524–30.
7. Overvad TF, Nielsen PB, Larsen TB, et al. Left atrial size and risk of stroke in patients in sinus rhythm. A systematic review. Thromb Haemost 2016;116(2):206–19.
8. Tandon K, Tirschwell D, Longstreth WT Jr, et al. Embolic stroke of undetermined source correlates to atrial fibrosis without atrial fibrillation. Neurology 2019;93(4):e381–7.
9. Mardigyan V, Verma A, Birnie D, et al. Anticoagulation management pre- and post-atrial fibrillation ablation: a survey of Canadian centres. Can J Cardiol 2013;29(2):219–23.
10. Lip GY, Proclemer A, Dagres N, et al. Periprocedural anticoagulation therapy for devices and atrial fibrillation ablation. Europace 2012;14(5):741–4.
11. Noseworthy PA, Yao X, Deshmukh AJ, et al. Patterns of anticoagulation use and cardioembolic risk after catheter ablation for atrial fibrillation. J Am Heart Assoc 2015;4:4.
12. Romero J, Cerrud-Rodriguez RC, Diaz JC, et al. Oral anticoagulation after catheter ablation of atrial fibrillation and the associated risk of thromboembolic events and intracranial hemorrhage: a systematic review and meta-analysis. J Cardiovasc Electrophysiol 2019;30(8):1250–7.
13. Karasoy D, Gislason GH, Hansen J, et al. Oral anticoagulation therapy after radiofrequency ablation of atrial fibrillation and the risk of thromboembolism and serious bleeding: long-term follow-up in nationwide cohort of Denmark. Eur Heart J 2015;36(5):307–314a.
14. Themistoclakis S, Corrado A, Marchlinski FE, et al. The risk of thromboembolism and need for oral anticoagulation after successful atrial fibrillation ablation. J Am Coll Cardiol 2010;55(8):735–43.
15. Nademanee K, Schwab MC, Kosar EM, et al. Clinical outcomes of catheter substrate ablation for high-risk patients with atrial fibrillation. J Am Coll Cardiol 2008;51(8):843–9.
16. Riley MP, Zado E, Hutchinson MD, et al. Risk of stroke or transient ischemic attack after atrial fibrillation ablation with oral anticoagulant use guided by ECG monitoring and pulse assessment. J Cardiovasc Electrophysiol 2014;25(6):591–6.
17. Zuern CS, Kilias A, Berlitz P, et al. Anticoagulation after catheter ablation of atrial fibrillation guided by implantable cardiac monitors. Pacing Clin Electrophysiol 2015;38(6):688–93.
18. Passman R, Leong-Sit P, Andrei AC, et al. Targeted anticoagulation for atrial fibrillation guided by

continuous rhythm assessment with an insertable cardiac monitor: the rhythm evaluation for anticoagulation with continuous monitoring (REACT.COM) pilot study. J Cardiovasc Electrophysiol 2016; 27(3):264–70.

19. Available at: http://grantome.com/grant/NIH/R34-HL113404-02#panel-publication. Accessed November 11, 2019.

20. Zado ES, Pammer M, Parham T, et al. As Needed" nonvitamin K antagonist oral anticoagulants for infrequent atrial fibrillation episodes following atrial fibrillation ablation guided by diligent pulse monitoring: a feasibility study. J Cardiovasc Electrophysiol 2019;30(5):631–8.

21. Available at: https://clinicaltrials.gov/ct2/show/NCT01959425. Accessed November 11, 2019.

22. Verma A, Ha ACT, Kirchhof P, et al. The optimal anticoagulation for enhanced-risk patients post-catheter ablation for atrial fibrillation (OCEAN) trial. Am Heart J 2018;197:124–32.

Moving?

Make sure your subscription moves with you!

To notify us of your new address, find your **Clinics Account Number** (located on your mailing label above your name), and contact customer service at:

Email: journalscustomerservice-usa@elsevier.com

800-654-2452 (subscribers in the U.S. & Canada)
314-447-8871 (subscribers outside of the U.S. & Canada)

Fax number: 314-447-8029

Elsevier Health Sciences Division
Subscription Customer Service
3251 Riverport Lane
Maryland Heights, MO 63043

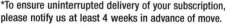
*To ensure uninterrupted delivery of your subscription, please notify us at least 4 weeks in advance of move.

ELSEVIER

Moving?

Make sure your subscription moves with you!

To notify us of your new address, find your Clinics Account Number (located on your mailing label above your name), and contact customer service at:

Email: journalscustomerservice-usa@elsevier.com

800-654-2452 (subscribers in the U.S. & Canada)
314-447-8871 (subscribers outside of the U.S. & Canada)

Fax number: 314-447-8029

Elsevier Health Sciences Division
Subscription Customer Service
3251 Riverport Lane
Maryland Heights, MO 63043

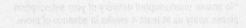

Printed and bound by CPI Group (UK) Ltd, Croydon, CR0 4YY

03/10/2024

01040307-0013